Essential Oils and Aromatherapy Bundle

The Beginner's Guide to Natural Healing Using the Power of Essential Oil

Essential Oils and Aromatherapy Bundle

The Beginner's Guide to Natural Healing Using the Power of Essential Oil

Natural Remedies for Health, Beauty, and Wellness Using This Ancient Medicine

Olivia Banks

Essential Oils and Aromatherapy Bundle: The Beginner's Guide to Natural Healing Using the Power of Essential Oil

Natural Remedies for Health, Beauty, and Wellness Using This Ancient Medicine

Copyright © 2018 Olivia Banks

Published by CAC Publishing LLC.

ISBN 978-1-948489-95-9 paperback

ISBN 978-1-948489-94-2 eBook

Table of Contents

Essential Oil for Beginners

The Ultimate Essential Oils Guide for Beginners

Essential Oil for Beginners

The Ultimate Essential Oils Guide for Beginners

Includes History, Benefits, Household Uses, Safety Tips, Essential Oils for Headaches, Sleep, Anxiety, and Other Ailments

Olivia Banks

CAC Publishing

Olivia Banks

ISBN: 978-1-948489-12-6

Introduction

Plant based oils and aromas have been used since time immemorial by thousands of communities and cultures across the world. They were even considered valuable products which could be used to: purchase luxurious items, pay dowry, settle disputes and offered as a gift to the gods; rivaling the likes of gold and silver. They have stood the test of time. The process of extracting oils from plants is something that has transformed and today it is much more efficient and cost effective. There is not much of a difference in terms of how various essential oils were being used in the past versus how they are being used today. The only change we've seen is that more uses have been developed for these oils.

The world of essential oils is so vast that more and more oils continue to be discovered as their usage expands. Often times it can be quite overwhelming as a beginner looking to get into this industry. *"The Ultimate Guide to Essential Oils"* aims to provide you with all the necessary information about essential oils in a detailed and easy to understand fashion. This book will help you identify the basic and most popular oils and their uses while gradually introducing you to more composite oils. You will learn how to create custom blends that work for you as well as the best ways to introduce their wonderful effects to your body. I hope that you will have fun and enjoy reading this book!

Chapter 1: History and Evolution

What are Essential Oils?

Essential oils are natural aromatic compounds found in the seeds, bark, stems, roots, flowers and other parts of plants gathered from around the world. While it is true they can be very fragrant, essential oils are extremely therapeutic. These natural oils are usually distilled from plants and are used most commonly for aroma therapy

Generally, these oils can be used in three different ways. The first one is known as **diffusion**. It involves the spreading of a type of oil into the air using a special device called a diffuser. Diffusers might be electrical devices you plug in or a sort of cup that holds essential oils and is then heated by a candle to diffuse the smell throughout the air.

One of the other ways to use an essential oil is the **topical** application meaning you are applying an essential oil right to your skin. However, some oils shouldn't be applied directly to your skin at all; while some should be diluted with other oils like coconut oil before it even touches your skin.

The other method is referred to as **ingestion**. Some people ingest essential oils whether taking a straight drop in their mouth or in a glass of water or even in their cooking. Extreme caution should be taken when ingesting essential oils as some can be very toxic. You should research and / or consult your doctor before ingesting any essential oil.

Essential oils are considered a dietary aide and provide vitality and well-being. They contain multifaceted naturally occurring compounds which makes them unique. These unique molecules allow essential oils to work with all the cells and tissues in the body.

It has been estimated that essential oils can be as much as 70 times more effective than dried herbs. As a matter of fact, one drop of peppermint is as potent as 28 cups or more of peppermint tea. Essential oils are immediately reactive in the body because their chemical structures are already in their most usable form.

Not all essential oils are alike. To be safe and effective, they must be pure and free from any alterations that would reduce their therapeutic benefit and their life sustaining properties.

In order to be most effective and beneficial, essential oils must be sourced in their native and often indigenous habitat.

Brief History and Timeline

Throughout history, people have used many forms of plant medicine; especially essential oils. Many believe that the Egyptians were the first to discover the benefits and therapeutic effects of these oils. As a matter of fact, essential oils were considered to be very valuable. Grave robbers often left the gold and jewels in the tombs and took only the oil. Over time, other cultures used essential oils for a variety of therapeutic treatments.

Many cultures around the world have used essential oils or aromatic oils as they were once called. While it may be quite difficult to pin point exactly when the use of essential oils began spreading, research into ancient civilization and societies have been able to give us a picture of just how popular these oils were in the past. Now, let us briefly examine some evidence of early use of essential oils.

France

So far, the earliest evidence of use of essential oils by human beings was found in a place called Lascaux in the Dordogne region of France. This region is covered by an extensive network of complex caves. Inside some of these caves are cave paintings that suggest the use of herb oils and medicinal plants in everyday life of the residents of that area. Carbon dating estimates the cave paintings to be at least 20,000 years old; meaning they were carved as far back as 18,000 B.C.E.

Egypt

Evidence along with recorded history of early Egyptians regarding use of essential oils is much more concrete. As far back as 5,000 B.C.E, Egyptians used aromatic oils and ointments for various purposes. As a matter of fact, at the time, they had made a name for themselves as experts in cosmetology and ointments; with their star herbal concoction called "Kyphi". It was used as medicine, incense and perfume and was made from a mixture of 16 ingredients.

The average citizen of Egypt used perfumed oils, resins, balsams, aromatic vinegars, spices and scented barks in their daily lives. Oils were extracted from plants to make pastes, powders, ointments, medicinal cakes as well as pills. Also used extensively during this period were: ashes and smoke from garlic, aniseed, grapes, watermelon and onion. However, it is worth noting that the use of aromatic oils was a privilege that was only reserved for priests; particularly at the height of the Egyptian Empire. It was viewed as a divine product that could only be handled by representatives of the gods.

To get a clearer picture, each deity had their own specific fragrance while the pharaohs also had their own special oils for various uses such as meditation and war. For purposes of preserving dead bodies, usually pharaohs and other high ranking royal family members, the early Egyptians used aromatic gums derived from cedar and myrrh. Evidence of their use has been traced to mummies found in recent times.

However, Egypt didn't always manufacture all the oils they used; they imported some – particularly cedar and cypress oils.

China

Use of essential oils in China was first recorded between the years 2697 B.C.E and 2597 B.C.E. Perhaps the most important piece of evidence with regards to this subject is the well documented journal called *"The Yellow Emperor's Book of Internal Medicine"* written during the reign of Emperor Huang Ti. Regarded as the oldest surviving medical book in China, it contains information on more than 300 herbs and their medicinal applications. To date, classic practitioners of eastern medicine still use it for research information.

India

A 3,000-year old branch of traditional Indian medicine known as *"Ayur Veda"* is very popular for its extensive use of essential oils. With an archive of more than 700 substances such as: myrrh, cinnamon, ginger and sandalwood in Vedic medicinal literature, traditional Indian medicine is regarded as one of the most comprehensive forms of traditional and alternative medicine.

Ayur Veda has been tried and tested thanks to its success in helping contain the spread of the Bubonic Plague by replacing some antibiotics that weren't working.

The use of aromatic oils was not just limited to medicinal purposes. Spiritual and philosophical outlook was also a major sphere of life for ancient Indians and these oils played a key role here as well.

Greece

Ancient Greek medicine (400 B.C.E to 500 B.C.E) contains a blend of ancient Egyptian medicine practices and the traditional Indian Ayur Veda, both of which are founded on essential oils. In ancient Greece, Hippocrates was commonly known as the *"Father of Medicine"*. He once said, *"I believe that a daily aromatic bath followed by a scented massage will promote good health"*. Under his advisement, soldiers often carried into battles ointments of myrrh to fight off infections. His literature contains documented effects of more than 300 plants such as marjoram, cumin, thyme and saffron.

Hippocrates was drawn to Ayurvedic medicine after Greek soldiers encountered it during their journeys with Alexander the Great and found it to be harmonious with Greek medicine. One of his many noble accomplishments was when he saved Athens from a deadly plague by fumigating the city with aromatics. To understand just how much of an influence and impact Hippocrates' work has had, all doctors today are required to take what is known as the *'Hippocratic Oath'*.

Europe

Use of essential oils for medicinal and spiritual purposes by the 14th Century was quite extensive across Europe. For instance, the knights during the crusades passed on knowledge of herbal medicine they had picked up from their travels in the Middle East. Also recorded in history books is how burning frankincense and pine in the streets during the Bubonic Plague helped contain the outbreak. More recently, in 1928, a French chemist called René-Maurice Gattefossé published the book "Aromatherapie" which describes in detail various essential oils and their healing capabilities.

Modern trends toward a more holistic approach to self-care and growing scientific validation of alternative health practices are driving a rediscovery of the profound health benefits of essential oils.

Evolution

The most well-known and recorded method of ancient extraction of essential oils is perhaps the method coined by ancient Egyptians. Now, since the process of using steam for distillation to extract essences was not invented back then, they had to use other techniques. One such method is called Enfleurage. It involves saturation of layers of fat with perfume by steeping flowers in the fat and replacing them when their perfume was spent. The flower petals are placed on a layer of glass that is spread with a layer of fat. What happens is that the volatile oil in the petals diffuses into the fat which is then collected and then oil is extracted from it using alcohol. This method is not used today because it is very expensive and time consuming. However, it worked for the ancient Egyptians and other ancient communities as well.

Today, the most commonly used methods for extraction of essential oils are:

- Steam distillation method
- Solvent extraction method

- Carbon dioxide extraction method
- Maceration process

Religious References of Essential Oils

There is a lot of reference to essential oils made in The Bible – both the Old and New Testament. Specifically mentioned are: myrrh, myrtle, frankincense, fir, spikenard, cinnamon and cedar wood. A well-known reference is one made regarding the birth of the child Christ during which he received gifts in the form of frankincense, myrrh and gold. Another reference of essential oils is made when Moses received the formula for holy anointing oil which included: olive oil, clove, cinnamon and myrrh.

The Holy Quran also makes reference to certain plants and plant extractions which were to be used as directed by Prophet Muhammad for medicinal purposes. They include: Onions (Basal), Hina (Henna), Grapes (Inab), Camphor (Kafoor), Date palm (Khajoor), Sweet Basil (Rehan), Figs (An-jeer) and many more.

Spiritual use of aromatic oils was not just limited to Christians and Muslims. As mentioned in the previous section, they were also used by ancient Egyptians, Jews, Indians as well as traditional African societies for spiritual purposes.

The World of Aromatherapy: Brief Introduction and Facts

Aromatherapy is the use of plant materials and plant oils to positively affect mood, psychological and / or physical well-being. In simple terms it comes down to: you smell nice things and it makes you feel good.

Aromatherapy has been around for thousands of years and basically involves your smell sense and different natural substances as a beneficial aid to your health and mental faculties.

So how is aromatherapy performed? Well, this is how:

- ✓ Directly inhaling essential oils through the nostrils from the bottle or off a cloth
- ✓ By diffusing one or a combination of essential oils into the surrounding air

- ✓ By rubbing the oils directly onto your skin
- ✓ By receiving a massage therapy using essential oils
- ✓ By soaking in an oil-infused bath

As you continue reading this book, you will understand the various kinds of essential oils and how you can use them to achieve the best results for your body and well-being.

Chapter 2: Health and Healing

Benefits of Essential Oils

Physical Health

Essential oils have been proven to support physical well-being time and time again. They can be used as part of a concoction or separately. Thousands of communities and millions of people across the world have used (and continue to use) the following essences and essential oils to help treat or reduce inflammation for certain physical ailments. Here are some of the most well-known and the physical ailments they can assist with:

Angelica Root Oil - Psoriasis, Dull skin, Water retention by the body, Gout and Toxin build up

Anise Oil - Flu, Bronchitis, Muscle aches, Rheumatism, Flatulence and Coughs

Basil Oil - Sinusitis, Gout, Bronchitis, Muscle aches, Insect bites, Rheumatism, Exhaustion, Flu and Coughs

Bay Leaf Oil - Poor circulation, hair Care, Neuralgia, Dandruff, Sprains and Oily Skin

Bay Laurel - Flu, Tonsillitis, Colds, Loss of appetite and Amenorrhea

Benzoin Oil - Chapped skin, Laryngitis, Amenorrhea, Flu and Colds

Bergamot Oil - Oily skin, Psoriasis, Acne, Boils, Cold sores and Halitosis

Bois de Rose (Rosewood Oil) - Oily skin, Scars, Acne, Colds, Sensitive skin, Stretch marks, Fever and Flu

Cajeput Oil - Sore throat, Muscle aches, Oily skin, Rheumatism, Sinusitis, Asthma and Bronchitis

Cardamom Oil - Halitosis, Loss of appetite and Coli

Carrot Seed Oil - Gout, Toxin build up and Eczema

Cedar Wood Atlas Oil - Dermatitis, Dandruff, Arthritis, Coughing, Bronchitis and Acne

Cedar Wood Oil - Dermatitis, Dandruff, Arthritis, Coughing, Bronchitis and Acne

German Chamomile Essence - Sores, Sprains, Rheumatism, Allergies, Colic Cuts, Hair care, Headaches, PMS, Strains, Dermatitis, Inflamed skin, Flatulence, Abscesses and Neuralgia

Roman Chamomile Essence - Sores, Sprains, Rheumatism, Allergies, Colic Cuts, Hair care, Headaches, PMS, Strains, Dermatitis, Inflamed skin, Flatulence, Abscesses and Neuralgia

Cinnamon Oil - Scabies, Flatulence, Constipation, Lice, Low blood pressure and Exhaustion

Citronella Essence - Oily skin, Fatigue, Headache, Excessive perspiration and Insect bites

Clary Sage Oil - Sore throat, Asthma, Amenorrhea, Labor pains and Coughing

Clove Bud Oil - Asthma, Sprains, Arthritis, Toothache, and Rheumatism

Coriander Oil - Nausea, Gout, Colic, Aches, Indigestion and Rheumatism

Cypress Oil - Hemorrhoids, Oily Skin, Excessive perspiration and Varicose veins

Elemi Oil - Wounds, Scars, Bronchitis, Coughing and Catarrh

Eucalyptus Globulous Oil - Sinusitis, Arthritis, Cold sores, Poor circulation, Flu and Fever

Fennel Oil - Toxin build up, Flatulence, Halitosis, Nausea and Cellulite

Frankincense - Stretch marks, Bronchitis, Coughing, Scars and Asthma

Galbanum Oil - Scars, Muscle aches, Bronchitis, Cuts, Sores, Lice, Acne and Boils

Geranium Oil - Lice, Oily skin, Acne and Cellulite

Ginger Oil - Nausea, Muscle ache, Arthritis and Poor circulation

Grapefruit Oil - Toxin build up, Cellulite and Dull skin

Helichrysum Oil - Boils, Wounds, Cuts, Acne, Burns, Abscesses and Eczema

Hyssop Oil - Sore throat, Bruises and Coughing

Jasmine Oil - Sensitive skin, Dry skin and Labor pains

Juniper Berry Oil - Gout, Toxin build up, Cellulite, Rheumatism and Hemorrhoids

Lavender Oil - Oily skin, Itchy skin, Headache, Cuts, Stretch marks, Acne, Flatulence, Allergies, Asthma, Insect bites, Insect repellant, Sprains, Colic Burns, Scabies and Scars

Lemon Oil - Oily skin, Varicose veins, Colds, Athlete's foot and Warts

Lemongrass Oil - Oily skin, Acne, Scabies, Athlete's foot, Excessive perspiration and Flatulence

Linden Blossom Oil - Scars, Spots, Oily skin, Headaches, Migraines and Wrinkles

Marjoram Oil - Sprains, Cramps, Muscle ache, Arthritis, Migraine and Neuralgia

Melissa Oil - Herpes, Shingles, Cold sores, Flu and Indigestion

Myrrh - Halitosis, Athlete's foot, Bronchitis, Ringworm and Amenorrhea

Myrtle - Coughs, Irritated skin and Asthma

Neroli - Stretch marks, Scars and Oily skin

Niaouli - Colds, Coughs, Sore throat, Bronchitis, Acne and Oily skin

Nutmeg Oil - Muscle ache, Constipation, Poor circulation, Nausea and Rheumatism

Bitter Orange Oil - Flatulence, Flu, Colds, Constipation, Dull skin and Bleeding gums

Oregano Oil - Respiration, Colds and Digestion

Parsley Oil - Kidney complications, Digestion, Congestion and Diuretic

Patchouli Oil - Oily skin, Dandruff, Eczema, Acne, Chapped skin, Dermatitis and Cellulite

Black Pepper Oil - Constipation, Detox, Muscle ache, Muscle cramps, Poor circulation and Arthritis

Peppermint Oil - Vertigo, Exhaustion, Fever, Flatulence, Nausea, Asthma, Scabies and Sinusitis

Petit-grain Oil - Insomnia and Rapid heartbeat

Pine Oil - Flu, Sinusitis, Colds and Congestion

Rose Oil - Eczema

Rosemary Oil - Muscle ache, Hair care, Gout, Neuralgia, Arthritis, rheumatism, Dandruff and Exhaustion

Sandalwood Oil - Urinary tract problems, Bronchitis, Oily skin and Strep throat

Spearmint Oil - Nausea, Headache, Asthma, Exhaustion, Scabies and Flatulence

Thyme Oil - Dermatitis, Arthritis, Bronchitis, Cuts and Laryngitis

Vetiver Oil - Oily skin, Muscle aches, Arthritis and Rheumatism

Violet Leaf Oil - Insomnia, Bronchitis, Poor circulation and Congestion

Yarrow Oil - Hypertension, Inflammation, Arthritis, Acne, Hair care and Insomnia

Ylang Ylang Oil - Palpitations, Hypertension and PMS symptoms

Emotional and Mental Health

Essential oils are also beneficial emotionally and mentally. Below I've noted benefits of various oils when it comes to reducing or resolving a number of emotional issues.

Angelica Root Oil - Stress and Nervousness

Anise Oil - Depression

Basil Oil - Exhaustion, Burnout and Fatigue

Bay Leaf Oil - Emotional exhaustion

Bay Laurel - Confidence booster

Benzoin Oil - Emotional insecurities

Bergamot Oil - Emotional insecurities, Anger, Anxiety, Depression, Fatigue and Confidence

Bois de Rose (Rosewood Oil) - Emotional imbalance and Depression

Cajeput Oil - Mental Fatigue and Emotional Confusion

Cardamom Oil - Guilt feelings, Stress and Shame

Carrot Seed Oil - Mood swings, Mental exhaustion, Stress and Anxiety

Cedar Wood Atlas Oil - Anxieties, Insecurities and Stress

Cedar Wood Oil - Anxieties, Insecurities and Stress

German Chamomile Essence - Anxieties, Insecurities, Depression, Loneliness and Stress

Roman Chamomile Essence - Irritability, Anxiety, Emotional Stress, Depression, Fear and Insomnia

Cinnamon Oil - Mental Concentration and Emotional and Mental Fatigue

Citronella Essence - Mind fog and Tension

Clary Sage Oil - Loneliness, Mental stress and Fear

Clove Bud Oil - Mental concentration and Depression

Coriander Oil - Irritability and Fatigue

Cypress Oil - Grief, Confidence issues and Mental concentration

Elemi Oil - Grief and Agitation

Eucalyptus Globulous Oil - Mental concentration

Fennel Oil - Emotional imbalance

Frankincense - Depression, Panic attacks, Anxiety, Loneliness, Grief, Emotional insecurities and Mental exhaustion

Galbanum Oil - Nervousness, Mood swings and Emotional rigidity

Geranium Oil - Anxiety, Emotional imbalance, Depression and Stress

Ginger Oil - Mental exhaustion and Burnout

Grapefruit Oil - Confidence issues, Stress, Fear and Depression

Helichrysum Oil - Loneliness, Grief and Panic Attacks

Hyssop Oil - Mental concentration and Nervousness

Jasmine Oil - Depression, Emotional fatigue, Stress, Confidence issues and Burnout

Juniper Berry Oil - Negative energy and Agitation

Lavender Oil - Panic attacks, Anxiety and Irritability

Lemon Oil - Memory issues and Fear

Lemongrass Oil - Emotional and mental confusion

Linden Blossom Oil - Stress and Tension

Marjoram Oil - Mood swings and PMS symptoms

Melissa Oil - Nervousness, Tension and Agitation

Myrrh - Emotional imbalance and Creativity

Myrtle - Depression, Addiction and Self-destructive tendencies

Neroli - Irritability, Anxiety, Stress and Panic attacks

Niaouli - Emotional concentration

Nutmeg Oil - Mental fatigue

Bitter Orange Oil - Depression, Confidence issues and Stress

Oregano Oil - Emotional insecurities

Parsley Oil - Emotional and mental rigidity

Patchouli Oil - Mental and emotional exhaustion and Stress

Black Pepper Oil - Emotional and mental fatigue and Anxiety

Peppermint Oil - Burnout, Mental concentration and Emotional fatigue

Petit-grain Oil - Panic attacks and Anxiety

Pine Oil - Depression, Nervousness and Exhaustion

Rose Oil - Panic attacks, Depression, Grief, Loneliness and Stress

Rosemary Oil - Mental exhaustion, Confidence issues, Burnout and Mental concentration

Sandalwood Oil - Stress, Irritability, Anxiety and Depression

Spearmint Oil - Depression and Mental and Emotional fatigue

Thyme Oil - Mental concentration

Vetiver Oil - Anger, Emotional insecurities, Grief and Stress

Violet Leaf Oil - Nostalgia obsession and Shyness

Yarrow Oil - Tension, Stress and Insomnia

Ylang Ylang Oil - Mood swings, Stress and Anger

Spiritual Health

Human beings have also incorporated essential oils and essences in prayers and spiritual journeys. Some of the oldest accounts of these have been recorded in The Bible and Holy Quran as well as historical accounts dating back to the Egyptian Empire and Ancient Indians which we explored in Chapter 1 of this book. Spiritual journeys are personal and vary from individual to individual and different essential oils speak out uniquely to different people. However, through extensive research, I was able to find that essential oils help in the following areas:

- ✓ Purification of the soul
- ✓ Promoting a harmonious environment
- ✓ Promoting love for one another
- ✓ Offering meaningful prayers while connecting to your higher power
- ✓ Harnessing the virtue of patience

Household Uses of Essential Oils

With seemingly endless choices of essential oils and their uses, often times, people get confused and overwhelmed as to what exactly to buy and how to use it. Now, around the house and for day to day activities, essential oils can work miracles. Here's how you can put your essential oil collection to work for your household purposes.

- ✓ You can deodorize the air around your house and in your fridge with lime oil and grapefruit oil.
- ✓ Get rid of that persistent pungent smell from your trash bin with geranium or lemon oil sprinkled into baking soda.
- ✓ Wipe dusty surfaces clean and stain by using orange oil, lemon oil or grapefruit oil.
- ✓ Make an insect repellant out of your peppermint oil, lavender oil, lemongrass oil, and citronella or rosemary oil.
- ✓ Clean your kids' sports outfit by adding tea tree oil and lemon oil to baking soda and warm water.
- ✓ Whip up peppermint patties for guests by using coconut oil, peppermint oil, dark chocolate and raw honey.

- ✓ Give scents to your washed clothes by adding a few drops of your favorite essence to the load in your washing machine.
- ✓ Make a DIY carpet cleaner powder by adding some tea tree oil to Borax.
- ✓ You can also use lemon oil mixed with water to wash fresh fruits and vegetables.
- ✓ Keep your shoes' odor at bay by infusing lemon oil, geranium oil, basil oil or lavender oil.
- ✓ Neutralize pet odor with a proper mixture of lavender oil or geranium with vinegar.
- ✓ Get rid of mites from your beddings by washing them with Eucalyptus oil mixed with water.
- ✓ Whip up a bunch of quick homemade recipes such as: mint tea and flavored lemon water, using your favorite essential oils.

Household uses of essential oil are practically limitless. Putting these oils to proper use will give you and your family the much needed calmness, comfort and tranquility living in a clean and peaceful environment.

Busting 5 Most Common Essential Oils Myths

Worldwide awareness of the fantastic healing properties of essential oils will continue to grow, but it is important that we dispel the misinformation about what these healing compounds are and what they can do. Much of the misinformation and myths involving essential oils are rooted in personal desire or corporate desire to sell more oils to unsuspecting people. So, let's set the record straight on some of the myths about essential oils.

Myth #1: Essential Oils Cures Everything for Everyone

In our collective effort to heal the world naturally, we must be careful not to get caught up in the one-size-fits-all fallacy. The success you may discover with one type of oil may not have the same result for your friend. We often see fallacious conclusions to explain this discrepancy with the following statements:

"You didn't pray hard enough or believe well enough"

"You must have received the bad batch of the oil"

"You didn't use this oil correctly"

"Essential oils simply don't work"

Our bodies respond differently to the complex compounds of essential oil. Where you find success with one type of essential oil, your friend might find the same success for the same condition with a completely different type of essential oil. Seek out every natural option to improve your health but be open to the fact that essential oils might not be the end-all fix for the condition you are targeting.

Myth #2: Essential Oils Labeled as "Therapeutic Grade" or "Clinical Grade" are of the Highest Quality

There is no governing body that certifies grades of essential oil. The quality behind an essential oil has more to its story that can be revealed by a GC-MS test

(Grade Chromatography-Mass Spectrometry). Therapeutic Grade and Clinical Grade are great examples but not an exhaustive list of marketing terms made up by certain companies to set their oils above that of the other companies. The companies producing the oil decides to label their oils with these terms; not a third party authority. As an individual user, you should be interested in what the company's position is on the quality of the oils they are selling.

Therefore, you should make plans to do a little more research and ask a few more questions about how the company produces their essential oils to get a clearer picture of the quality rather than shopping for oil simply based on a company's chosen marketing term.

Myth #3: The Best Place to Apply Essential Oils are the Soles of the Feet

Massage Today and Aromatherapy United debunked this popular practice. Dermatology science shows that our stratum corneum (the outermost layer of skin) is the thickest on the soles of our feet which makes it more difficult for essential oils to penetrate cell membranes. While it is true that our feet are very porous when compared to the rest of our body, it is also true that these pores are mostly sweat glands that are not a reliable delivery method to the blood. Alternatively, the stratum corneum on the arms, back, legs and abdomen are much thinner and much more effective locations for penetration of essential oils.

Myth #4: With Essential Oils, You Always Get What You Pay For

This phrase is commonly used by companies or individuals selling higher price oils. While it can be true that you get what you pay for, it is also true that you can overpay for what you get. If you are willing to pay a higher price for a brand that others can't afford or you simply aren't willing to overpay, it is important to understand that higher priced oil is not always an indication that the oil is of higher quality. Price considerations should certainly be part of your evaluation process when deciding what brands of oil you would like to purchase. However, don't fall victim to the misconception that the price of the oil automatically makes that oil higher-quality.

Myth #5: Best Quality Essential Oils Never Deteriorate or Expire

If it were possible to store essential oils in a completely oxygen-free atmosphere, then there could possibly be some truth to this myth. However, in the world we live in, everything oxidizes and breaks down with time – even 100% pure essential oils. Nonetheless, proper care of your essential oil bottles will allow your oils to last for years. This should include storing your oils in a dark, cool place away from direct sunlight and keeping your lids tight when not in use.

Chapter 3: A Word for Beginners

Keep Out of Eyes, Ears and Open Wounds (Burns, Cuts and Bruises)

Avoid getting oil in your eyes or ears. You'll want to avoid contact with any sensitive areas or wounds on the body; so make sure you wash your hands after applying the oils. If you happen to get a little oil in your eyes, flush it out with olive, vegetable or fractionated coconut oil. To flush your eyes with oil you can use a tissue and gently wipe the area. Your natural reaction might be to use water; however, keep in mind that oil and water don't mix. Using water might actually make things worse.

Always Read the Label

Be sure to look at the oil's label and review the provided product guide for usage and directions. Many oils can be used internally, topically and aromatically; however, not all of the oils can be used with all three application methods. You'll also want to note the provided sensitivity chart and make sure you are diluting the oil properly. If you have sensitive skin, you might want to keep some carrier oil handy when trying the oil for the first time.

Avoid Topical Usage of Citrus Oils in Direct Sunlight

Avoid using citrus oils topically when going into direct sunlight. This is because citrus oils can be photosensitive and can cause discoloration of the skin. Even using a tanning bed and using the citrus oils topically should be avoided.

Internal Consumption

Not all essential oils can be consumed internally. Typically, oils safe for internal consumption will be labeled by the FDA as GRAS (generally recognized as safe). Also, they will ordinarily come with a supplement facts box with dietary supplement, warnings and instructions.

Usage when Pregnant

It is advisable that you consult your doctor before using any essential oil when pregnant or under a doctor's care. Depending on your health condition, your physician will be able to properly advise you on what essential oils you can use and how to use them.

Remember that because essential oils are quite potent, a little goes a long way. You only need a few drops to experience the incredible benefits that come with their usage.

Ways to Use Essential Oils

As you already know by now, uses of essential oils are endless. Application of these oils can be done in a number of ways which vary based on the type of oil, the purpose for which it is being used as well as the effects of the oil on human skin. Without further ado, let us consider the following types of applications.

Skin Application

Due to their fat soluble nature, essential oils are almost immediately absorbed by the skin when applied. However, most people like to mix and dilute them with a neutral carrier oil such as coconut oil or sweet almond oil. More about carrier oils will be addressed in the next sub-topic. A common concern when using carrier oils is that they tend to go rancid therefore choice of carrier oils, for most people, is based on its smell, texture and sensitivities. The wrists, feet, behind the ears and temples are the most popular areas of application.

Simple Inhalation

This method involves pouring a few drops of your favorite oil onto the palm of your hands, rubbing them gently and briefly and then inhaling. Alternatively, you can pour a few drops on a tissue and inhale. For beginners, a couple of drops are enough to avoid any reactions or sensitivities.

Steam Inhalation

For steam inhalation, boil about 3 cups of water, pour into a bowl and add a few drops of your favorite oil. Now, place your nose about 10 inches from the bowl, cover your head with a cloth or towel and gently inhale the steam. You'd be surprised how relaxing this can become.

Essential Oil Diffuser

There are different types of electronic diffusers. They are convenient because all you have to do is feed a few drops of your favorite oil into the diffuser, turn it on and circulate in your room. Electronic diffusers are pretty simple to use and maintain.

Application through Baths

One of the most relaxing ways to unwind after a long or busy day is by soaking your body in a bath. Essential oils take this experience to a whole new level. Normally, you would use salts, such as Epsom salt, as the base to ensure that the oil you are adding dissolves properly for the best results. Remember not to use any chemically produced soap(s) during this relaxing bath time.

Aromatherapy Massage

For aromatherapy massage purposes, essential oils are mixed with neutral-smelling carrier oils such as grape seed oil or sweet almond oil. Measurements vary but anything in the neighborhood of a ratio of 20 drops of essential oil to an ounce of carrier oil should work just fine.

Carrier Oils

Carrier oils are a naturally derived vegetable oil of neutral smell. They are obtained from the fatty portion of a plant. Unlike essential oils, carrier oils are not volatile; making them perfect as a dilution medium. In a way, you could describe carrier oils as the indispensable companion of topically applied essential oils. Some of the most common types of carrier oils include:

- Coconut oil
- Olive oil
- Sweet almond oil
- Grapeseed oil
- Castor oil
- Flaxseed oil
- Jojoba oil
- Avocado oil
- Apricot kernel oil
- Black seed oil

Because they are high in fat, carrier oils have a limited shelf life which varies from six months to one year. To get maximum shelf life, carrier oils should be stored in an air tight container and in a dark cool place.

You can use carrier oils to make your own blends. If you have smaller vials, you can add some carrier oil to it along with a mixture of your essential oils to make your own custom blends. Carrier oils can also be used as massage oils by adding about 15 to 25 drops of essential oil to an ounce of carrier oil such as coconut oil.

Carrier oils come in handy if you accidentally apply essential oil in a sensitive part of your skin or body such as the eyes; since washing it out with water will make things worse.

Best 5 Essential Oils to Buy Under $100

There are tons of essential oils out there with numerous applications as well as varying price ranges. As a beginner, the information alone can get quite overwhelming. There is no doubt that essential oils have benefits, but that does not mean that every dealer or supplier of these products sell them at fair market price. Granted, there's a lot that goes into determining prices for different oils. Factors like the cost of distillation and availability of the parent plant, among others, play a key role in setting the price. That said, for beginners looking to buy good essential oils under $100, the following should be easily available:

- ✓ Lavender Oil
- ✓ Peppermint Oil
- ✓ Lemon Oil
- ✓ Frankincense

Finding a Good Supplier

It is no secret that essential oils continue to rise in popularity. They are much more readily available than they were, say, three decades ago. Many brands are popping up every year which also comes with an increase in unscrupulous suppliers. So, how do you maneuver this market without getting swindled? Well, before choosing any supplier, take into account the following:

Consider the Supplier's Pricing of Essential Oils

If the price looks too good to be true, it probably is. A lot of factors affect the final price of essential oils. The distillation process of extracting the oil is quite expensive as it is. Add to that the availability of the base plant and the physical and chemical properties of the oil and you can begin to understand why oils are priced differently. For example, at least 260 pounds of rose blossoms are needed to produce an ounce of rose oil. This should tell you that rose oil can't be cheap. A little research into a product you are interested in can go a long way in helping you decide whether you purchase it from supplier X or supplier Y.

Research on the Products' Purity and Testing

Since there is no standardized test for essential oil carried out by an independent third party, the issue of purity often gets a little tricky. As a general rule, make a point of finding out what purity tests the suppliers' brands perform and how they do it. Purity can be affected by seasons as well as where the plants grow.

A brand that explains to its customers, in detail, the extensive tests they carry out on their products and provide some sort of evidence for this builds a lot more trust. Also, as an essential oil user, you should check out reviews by past users of the same brand to help you make a decision.

Chapter 4: Essential Oils and Their Uses

The Top 50 Essential Oils

As you already know, essential oils come from plants. Every plant has its own unique aroma and therapeutic benefits, so it is only logical that the number of essential oils be in the hundreds, if not thousands. Naturally, this presents a challenge to many people when it comes to choosing essential oils to address different concerns. I did extensive research in the various essential oils available out there and came up with a shortlist of the top 53 most popular essential oils based on their multifold uses, availability, affordability and effectiveness. You should know that the following is just a list of the essential oils. The next chapter will discuss them in much more detail with respect to their multiple uses.

Basil Oil	Bergamot Oil	Cardamom Oil
Carrot Seed Oil	Cassia Oil	Cedar Wood Oil
Cilantro Oil	Cinnamon Oil	Clary Sage Oil
Clove Oil	Cypress Oil	Eucalyptus Oil
Fennel Oil	Frankincense Oil	Geranium Oil

German Chamomile Oil	Ginger Oil	Grapefruit Oil
Helichrysum Oil	Jasmine Oil	Jojoba Oil
Juniper Oil	Lavender Oil	Lemon Oil
Lemongrass Oil	Lime Oil	Marjoram Oil
Melaleuca Oil	Myrrh Oil	Neroli Oil
Oregano Oil	Palmarosa Oil	Patchouli Oil
Peppermint Oil	Pine Oil	Pomegranate Seed Oil
Roman Chamomile Oil	Rose Oil	Rosehip Oil
Rosemary Oil Sweet	Sandalwood Oil	Orange Oil
Tangerine Oil	Tarragon Oil	Tea Tree Oil
Thyme Oil	Turmeric Oil	Vetiver Oil
White Fir Oil	Wild Orange Oil	Wintergreen Oil
Yarrow Oil	Ylang-Ylang Oil	

Chapter 5: Best 3 in 10 Categories

Top 3 Essential Oils for Energy and Vitality

Peppermint Essential Oil

Peppermint essential oil has many uses, especially in terms of its shear medicinal value. Its active ingredient is menthol, which is found in high concentrations. This makes peppermint essential oil one of the strongest natural antibacterial, anti-fungal and anti-viral oils. Its strong, invigorating, minty aroma makes it excellent for boosting both mental and physical vitality. It has been used to boost concentration, fight fatigue and improve exercise performance.

How to Use Peppermint Essential Oil

There are three ways in which you can use peppermint essential oil to boost energy and vitality. They are as follows:

- Combine 1 drop of peppermint oil and 1 drop rosehip oil; rub them together and gently apply under your nose, base of your neck or shoulders.
- Add some to your diffuser and turn it on when you are studying or working on a project. It will help you concentrate and stay alert.
- You can also just inhale it directly. Ideally, you would do this before your workouts to help prevent lethargy while also giving you the energy and drive you need.

Eucalyptus Essential Oil

The main compound found in eucalyptus oil is cineole. It is a powerhouse of healing properties and has been found to feature antioxidant, anti-inflammatory and analgesic properties. Thanks to its multipurpose nature, many researchers have been drawn to study it. Findings from a 2010 study led to eucalyptus oil being described as an "immune-stimulator" with the capabilities of boosting energy levels in the body.

How to Use Eucalyptus Essential Oil

- Apply topically by rubbing a few drops of the oil on your wrists, muscles and temple after a long day. The tingling effect has a surprisingly strong calming effect.
- Add a few drops to your diffuser and let the menthol molecules provide an energizing aromatherapy.
- Add some drops to your shower to relieve the fatigue that comes with a cold. It will also uplift your mood.
- Direct inhalation from the bottle will provide you with an instant energy wake-me-up.

Ginger Essential Oil

When you are short on sleep and looking for something to jumpstart your mojo, ginger essential oil is your buddy. This spicy oil is great for maintaining energy levels, fighting feelings of sluggishness and revitalization.

How to Use Ginger Essential Oil

- You can inhale it directly from the bottle. Its hot aroma not only elevates your energy levels, it also fights off feelings of nausea or morning sickness – whether you are hungover or pregnant. For those interested in weight loss or maintaining a diet, this oil is known to reduce cravings and appetite.

- For topical application, add about 3 drops of ginger oil to some carrier oil such as Moringa oil and rub on your hands and feet. Once it is absorbed into the bloodstream, your vitality increases, senses become stimulated and overall energy is boosted.

Top 3 Essential Oils for Anxiety and Mental Health

Lavender Essential Oil

Lavender essential oil has a very fresh and floral aroma which is quite calming and relaxing. Referred to as an "adapt-o-gen", lavender essential oil is one of the most ideal picks for enhancing mood. Its nature as a mood enhancer makes it good for reducing stress, insomnia and calming agitation. There is growing scientific evidence that suggests topical application of anxiety-relieving essential oils is the most effective. Lavender oil has been found to enter the bloodstream within just a few minutes of rubbing on the skin.

How to Use Lavender Essential Oil

- Rub a few drops onto your palm and inhale directly. The oil penetrates to the center of emotions – also known as the amygdala – providing instant relaxation. Use it in high-stress areas such very crowded areas or in the office.

- Rub a few drops into your temples to ease tension and relieve headaches.

- Add a couple of drops in hot water to make a lavender herbal tea. It is very soothing and relaxing.

Cedar Wood Essential Oil

Cedar wood oil is yet another essential oil known for its stress relieving and calming properties. Once it penetrates the bloodstream, the aroma triggers the release of serotonin – a chemical that stabilizes mood in the brain. Serotonin can also be converted to melatonin to promote calmness and regulate sleep patterns; so, in effect, cedar wood essential oil is also a natural sedative.

How to Use Cedar Wood Essential Oil

- You can either rub a few drops on a handkerchief or the palm of your hands and inhale; or just inhale directly from the bottle.
- Rub some drops onto your neck or above your eyebrows to relieve tension.
- You can also, add some to your diffuser and let it waft through the air covering the whole room.

Grapefruit Essential Oil

Grapefruit essential oil is another type of citrus-based oil whose aroma is refreshing, uplifting and clarifying. The fruit itself has almost similar effects to lime. This stress-buster oil alleviates depression, mental fatigue and headaches resulting from stress. A simple whiff can go a long way in transforming your whole day for the better.

How to Use Grapefruit Essential Oil

- Using a diffuser to diffuse grapefruit oil aroma is perhaps the best way to tap into its effectiveness. Add a few drops in your diffuser and let it fill your room with anxiety-relieving aroma.

- You can also apply it topically. Along with some carrier oil such as jojoba or grapeseed oil, add a few drops to a cotton pad and gently rub onto your wrists and neck.

- Add some drops to your shower and cover the drain. As the water falls on your body, inhale deeply to enjoy its anxiety-relieving benefits.

Top 3 Essential Oils for Haircare

Rosemary Essential Oil

Rosemary essential oil is another multipurpose oil whose powerful effects are only matched by its fresh minty and woodsy scent; as Up Nature puts it: *"Rosemary's aroma is instantly youthful and deliciously herbaceous"*.

When it comes to haircare, rosemary oil is one of the most popular essential oils. It has a lot of antioxidants which stimulate hair follicles and prevent graying and thinning of hair. If you are struggling with an itchy scalp, rosemary oil can provide a great relief for dandruff while clearing pores. It also tones down the production of sebum which helps a lot with oily scalps.

How to Use Rosemary Essential Oil for Haircare

Heat about 3 to 4 tablespoons of olive oil over medium heat and blend in about a dozen drops of rosemary essential oil a few minutes later. Once thoroughly mixed, pour this oil treatment over your head and rub into your scalp. Dip a towel in hot water and wrap your hair with it and leave it for half an hour before shampooing it out. Make a point of doing this once a month and your hair will transform for the better.

Clary Sage Essential Oil

Of all sages, the clary sage is probably the most versatile. It has a distinct murky aroma; however, what makes it a good fit for hair care is its phytoestrogen content that is known to prevent, and in some cases reverse, premature balding. If you are suffering from excess dandruff production, clary sage oil can help to normalize your scalp's production of oil. It is not ideal for use when you are pregnant since it is known to induce contractions.

How to Use Clary Sage Essential Oil

If you intend to use clary sage oil to promote hair growth, blend equal parts of the oil and jojoba oil then rub it into your scalp. Give it about half an hour before shampooing it out.

Patchouli Essential Oil

Because patchouli has a very strong aroma, it is recommended that you use it in small amounts. This deep, earthy and sensual oil has antiseptic and anti-inflammatory properties which make it ideal for treating skin irritations. With patchouli essential oil, dandruff and eczema can quickly become a thing of the past. Hair loss brought by eczema can also be resolved in the process.

How to Use Patchouli Essential Oils

Blend together 1 part patchouli oil, 2 parts rosemary oil and 3 parts argan oil. Take this blend and massage it generously and deeply into your scalp and leave it for a couple of hours before shampooing it out.

Top 3 Essential Oils for Skincare, Aging and Acne

Frankincense Essential Oil

Frankincense essential oil promotes skin cell regeneration, meaning it prevents aging of the skin, making users look much more youthful. It also heals scars while reducing the appearance of wrinkles and lines.

How to Use Frankincense Essential Oils

Using this oil before you go to sleep at night helps the skin rejuvenate much faster while you sleep. Take a couple of drops of frankincense and blend it together with almond oil then apply it to your already cleansed and moisturized face. This blend can serve as a night mask. In case you made more than enough, you can store the excess blend in a dark glass container for future use.

Geranium Essential Oil

Geranium essential oil contains a lot of antioxidants which help fight signs of aging. The antioxidants work by fighting off the free radicals that your skin is exposed to on a daily basis. Thanks to its astringent properties, geranium oil can normalize oil production of the skin. This makes it an ideal choice for people struggling with oily skin. It makes the skin look more youthful by reducing the appearance of large, open pores.

How to Use Geranium Essential Oil

Geranium controls excess oil and breakouts thereby giving life to your skin. You can use it as a moisturizer. An ideal blend can be made mixing 1 part geranium oil with 5 parts jojoba oil that you apply as a primer before using your makeup.

Carrot Seed Essential Oil

Carrot seed oil reverses the harsh effects that occur on your skin when it is exposed to unhealthy environmental conditions over a long period of time. Before you leave the house, apply a few drops of this oil mixed with your favorite carrier oil. It helps maintain the youthful glow of your skin for longer periods of time.

How to Use Carrot Seed Essential Oil

Mix a few drops of carrot seed oil with some carrier oil such as jojoba oil and apply it to your skin. If you have oily skin, make a toner by adding some drops of carrot seed oil and apricot kernel oil to some rosewater and spray it on your face before applying your moisturizer.

Top 3 Essential Oils for Sleep and Relaxation

Roman Chamomile Essential Oil

Chamomile, in general, is quite popular for fighting insomnia; however, the Roman Chamomile is perhaps the strongest of all of them. Chamomile is an ancient herb that has therapeutic properties that relax the body and mind, hence acting as a sedative. So it comes as no surprise that it is a common pick for treating stress and nervous tension as well. In addition, its sweet and comforting scent has been found to treat hysteria and insomnia.

How to Use Roman Chamomile Essential Oil

- Add a few drops to the palm of your hands or a handkerchief and inhale deeply. You can also just inhale directly from the bottle.
- Add about 2 drops to a cup of black tea for that soothing feeling before you go to bed.

Bergamot Essential Oil

Bergamot essential oil is citrus-based and has one of the most pleasant smells of all essential oils. Recent studies have now confirmed what was believed that this oil greatly reduces anxiety and improves mood. What it does is cuts down the amount of cortisol in the saliva, giving it some sedative properties. By doing this, you get to spend more time in the restorative stage of sleep.

How to Use Bergamot Essential Oil

- Take a few drops of this oil, rub on the palm of your hands then cover your nose with your hands as you inhale deeply.
- For topical application, rub some of this oil on the back of your neck or temples before going to bed.

Lavender Essential Oil

There is no doubt that lavender oil is a powerhouse when it comes to multi-fold uses. It consistently features among the top and most popular choices of essential oils for various uses. It is made up of esters and alcohols that have therapeutic properties, such as relaxation. True lavender essential oil reigns supreme over other forms of lavender oil such as spike lavender and lavandin oils. It calms nerves, reduces the effects of asthma, improves digestion and relieves headaches; laying all the groundwork for a good night's sleep.

How to Use Lavender Essential Oil

- Rub a few drops onto your palm and inhale directly. The oil penetrates to the center of emotions – also known as the amygdala – providing instant relaxation. Use it in high-stress areas such very crowded areas or in the office.
- Rub a few drops into your temples to ease tension and relieve headaches.
- Add a couple of drops in hot water to make a lavender herbal tea. It is very soothing and relaxing.

Top 3 Essential Oils for Happiness and Mood

Ylang Ylang Essential Oil

The flower of this oil have an incredibly sweet and floral aroma that reduces the negative thoughts associated with depression and mood swings. Ylang ylang has already been seeing usage in mainstream and high-end perfume brands like Chanel. A recent study described this oil as, *"a relief for depression and stress in humans"*. It reduces stress levels, uplifts spirits and promotes happiness and calmness.

How to Use Ylang Ylang Essential Oil

- Apply topically by rubbing a few drops on your neck, wrists, and feet or behind your ears.

Sandalwood Essential Oil

Sandalwood is often found in incense. It has a woody, warm and calming aroma which helps clear your mind and help with meditation. The oil's scent is regarded as a strong emotional balancer thanks to its effect on the brain's limbic system. Not only does it enhance sleep quality through its sedative properties, it also reduces the feelings of depression.

How to Use Sandalwood Essential Oil

- You can inhale directly from its bottle or rub some onto the palm of your hands and inhaling.
- Add about 6 drops of this oil to 2 drops of rose oil and blend with jojoba oil then use this new blend to massage your wrists, feet and back.

Basil Essential Oil

Basil oil is very high in vitamin C and antioxidants which are known to calm the nerves and reduce inflammation. While Depression and happiness are polar opposites, Basil is known to help with both. Basil oil revitalizes energy levels, alleviates chronic fatigue and promotes calmness; all of which work against depression. This lays the foundation for a good mood (and happiness along the way).

How to Use Basil Essential Oil

- In your diffuser, add 3 parts basil oil to 1 part peppermint oil. The aroma will instantly uplift your mood and revitalize your energy.

Top 3 Essential Oils for Balancing Hormones

Thyme Essential Oil

Thyme oil boosts the production of progesterone in the body. So how does this help? Well, low progesterone levels in the body have been linked to infertility, depression and PCOS (polycystic ovarian syndrome). There is a well-documented study about this in the *'Proceedings of the Society of Experimental Biology and Medicine'*. Because it is a natural hormone balancer, it is preferred by many people over synthetic hormone replacement therapies.

Clary Sage Essential Oil

Clary sage essential oil is another type of oil with significant benefits to the body in terms of hormone balance. It reduces cortisol levels in the body thereby alleviating stress. It also improves thyroid hormone levels and balances out estrogen production in the body. The dangers hormonal imbalance poses to the body are endless, and with clary sage essential oil, you can avoid conditions like PCOS, cancers, chronic stress and infertility.

How to Use Clary Sage and Thyme Essential Oils

- Add 20 to 30 drops of clary sage oil to 20 to 30 drops of thyme essential oil and blend it with an ounce of primrose oil. Store this blend in a dark glass container from which you will be rubbing about 5 drops around your neck twice every week.

Sandalwood Essential Oil

Sandalwood balances out testosterone levels in both men and women. It has also been found to be a natural aphrodisiac. You can improve your libido and balance out your T-hormones with this oil.

How to Use Sandalwood Essential Oil

- Mix some coconut oil with sandalwood oil and rub it on different parts of the body. This will allow them to be absorbed into the body through the skin.

Top 3 Essential Oils for Gut Health and Digestion

Oregano Essential Oil

Oregano oil contains potent antibacterial, anti-fungal and anti-parasitic healing compounds making it one of the most powerful essential oils for digestion. It has been found to kill off pathogenic gut bacteria that live in the digestive system. Its active compound is called carvacrol which kills yeast and other harmful bacteria. Because it is so strong, it is only recommended for use when in distress to get regular digestion back on track.

How to Use Oregano Oil

- For digestive issues or viral infections, dilute a drop of this oil in 500 ml of water and drink it (make sure to check with your doctor before doing this).

Peppermint Essential Oil

This is a fragrant, stimulating and refreshing type of oil that is widely used for digestive issues. It also eases common nausea, indigestion, and gas while stimulating your digestive process.

How to Use Peppermint Essential Oil

- Add a drop or two in a vegetarian gel capsule and take daily or as needed.
- You can also blend it with your pre-workout drink for an energizing start or wind down after your workout with your favorite shake.

Ginger Essential Oil

The root of ginger has been used for centuries, and continues to be used, in kitchens all over the world for its ability to reduce symptoms of common stomach upset including nausea, bloating and gas. The oil extracted from it is used to stimulate digestion and sooth the gut.

How to Use Ginger Essential Oil

- Inhale some directly out of the bottle or put some in your diffuser. The vapors carry active chemical molecules into your body through the nose. These chemicals stimulate your nasal cavity sending signals directly to your central nervous system – the system by which digestion is governed.

Top 3 Essential Oils for Headaches, Injury and Pain Management

Chamomile Essential Oil

Chamomile's analgesic properties are very useful when treating headaches and neuralgia, along with muscle and joint pains. It can also be used to relieve abdominal pain brought by bloating. While German Chamomile is preferred when handling inflammatory conditions, Roman Chamomile is ideal in soothing abdominal discomfort.

How to Use Chamomile Essential Oil

- Use chamomile oil with a diffuser or apply topically to the affected area after diluting with some carrier oil.

Eucalyptus Essential Oil

Eucalyptus oil is a powerful decongestant with anti-inflammatory properties that contribute to pain relief from sinus congestion and muscle injuries. It is quite strong; therefore, it should be diluted with some carrier oil when applying on the skin. You can use it raw when used to treat insect stings and bites.

How to Use Eucalyptus Essential Oil

- Blend the oil with other Essential Oils such as Lavender to enhance its effects.
- Use in your bath water by dropping a few drops of the oil in it.
- You can also use as a lotion and rub it lightly on affected areas.

Peppermint Essential Oil

The highly refreshing smell of the oil comes from the active ingredient menthol – a major component of the oil. It has been used to relieve stomachaches, indigestion and nausea. When used topically, it relaxes muscles in the lower back, reduces tension headaches and pain due to fibromyalgia.

How to Use Peppermint Essential Oil

- Mix a few drops of this oil with a teaspoonful of some carrier oil. Apply the blend topically to the affected area, or the temples in case of a headache. Make sure the oil doesn't come in contact with your eyes.

Top 3 Essential Oils for Cleaning Your Home

Tea Tree Essential Oil

Tea tree oil is quite strong in killing germs, viruses and bacteria, and that is why it is a common ingredient in hand wipes and hand soaps. It can also be used as a bug repellant and an air freshener that gets rid of musty smells around your house. Not many essential oils have their antifungal and antiseptic properties off the charts quite like tea tree essential oil and for these reasons, it makes the list of the best oils for home cleaning.

How to Use Tea Tree Essential Oil

- Add a couple of teaspoons of this oil to two cups of water in a clean spray bottle to make a cleaner for moldy and dusty areas.
- Make a solution of water and mild soap and add a few drops of tea tree essential oil to it. Use the mixture to mop your floor.

Lemon Essential Oil

This oil is popular and preferred for its light and clean scent. Naturally antibacterial and antiviral, lemon is commonly used to degrease stubborn stains as well as make the air fresher for longer.

How to Use Lemon Essential Oil

- Lemon oil can be used in a myriad of different ways. You can combine it with olive oil to make for a natural wood or leather polish. You can mix it with other essential oils, such as lavender oil and tea tree oil, along with some alcohol, to make for a powerful house cleaning liquid.

- Add a few drops of this oil to your laundry detergent to brighten your white clothes and give them a fresh scent.

Wild Orange Essential Oil

Wild orange oil has many of the properties that lemon oil has with one of the few differences being that it has more of a 'happy' scent. It is a powerful grease remover, germ killer and air freshener. Just like lemon oil, wild orange oil also has a ton of uses and can be used both in combination with other oils or just by itself.

- Use a couple of drops to lift grease or glue from surfaces.
- Combine about a dozen drops with 1/4 cup castile soap and water to wipe down stovetops and counters.

Chapter 6: Fun with Oils

How to Use Essential Oils

Air Freshener Spray

It is hard to keep up with the number of home fragrance products available today. From scented sprays and oil diffusers to incense and plug-in room deodorizes, the industry has it all. The problem is that a lot of these products are filled with chemicals and toxins that are harmful to our bodies. A few drops of some highly concentrated essential oil can provide your home with the much needed sweet and fresh fragrance. For a homemade air freshener spray, all you need are: a clean empty spray bottle, some water, your favorite essential oil and a bit of undiluted alcohol such as vodka. The most commonly used essential oils in air fresheners sprays include: lavender, lemon, lime, rosemary, clary sage, clove and orange oils.

Bath Salts

You have probably heard of the soothing effects of a lavender essential oil bath or a peppermint essential oil bath. These baths offer a wonderful destressing, pain relieving, skin softening and relaxing feeling after a long hard day. These baths can also be used to treat bacterial infections. Oil and water do not mix; therefore, just adding some essential oil to your bath won't help much. In fact, if anything, it may irritate or burn your skin. You can mix it with a carrier oil first to negate the chances of irritation, but may still not mix properly with water. What people usually do is mix essential oil with some bath salts first so that it is able to fully disperse and infuse in the bath.

Add about 10 to 20 drops of oil, such as lavender or rosemary, to your favorite bath salts before infusing them in a water bath. The most common bath salts used with oils include: dead sea salt, Epsom salt and sea salt.

Candles

The idea behind burning scented candles is usually to eliminate foul odors in the room, create a more festive and welcoming atmosphere or for aromatherapy purposes such as uplifting the spirit and calming your mind. Making your own candles is as inexpensive as it is easy. These scented candles can also make for a good gift to your loved ones. Depending on the purpose you want to achieve, choose an essential oil that fits you. You can refer to the previous chapter in the uses of various oils.

Typically, the recommended ratio is an ounce of oil to a pound of wax but you can tweak it and see what works for you. It should be noted that since candles involve the oils coming into contact with direct heat, there is a possibility that you may get very little scent because the heat destroys the oils. Candles are not the most effective way to disperse wonderful fragrances around the house, but you can always try and see how it comes out.

Gel Sprays

Essential oils can provide a natural and cost-effective way to care for your dreadlocks. The most common blends being used today for gel sprays feature essential oils such as: tea tree oil, lavender oil, rosemary oil and peppermint oil mixed with a base such as Aloe Vera gel. Organic Aloe Vera is far better than its synthetic counterpart and it can be used to treat or relieve the following conditions.

- Burns
- Fungus
- Scalp itchiness
- Eczema
- As a hand sanitizer

Besides Aloe Vera, other bases used for making a DIY gel spray include: rich creams, lotions and heavy butters.

Humidifier

Diffusing essential oils in your house creates a pleasant scent, uplifts or calms your mood, cleanses the air, heals physical infirmities and balances emotions. Most diffusers use cold air to break down the particles of the essential oil which means the integrity of the oil is maintained. Humidifiers, on the other hand, use warm air which can damage the oil's particles thereby compromising its therapeutic properties. Also, because humidifiers run constantly, your body is not given the time to absorb the dispersed oil. Some essential oils such as citrus-based oils have been found to break down plastics, which can damage your humidifier in the long run. For these reasons it is not always advisable to use humidifiers to disperse essential oil.

Massage Oils

Aromatherapy massage provides a remarkable synergy that not only relieves stress and tension, but also boosts the general well-being of someone. Custom massage oils are commonly made by combining essential oils and carrier oils. There are a million recipes available for aromatherapy massage oils. If scent is huge deal breaker for you, make a point of sampling scents of different essential oils and carrier oils first so that you can get a sense of what the finished product will smell like. When mixing oils, do it one step at a time and sample the resulting scent. Keep track of the quantities or ratios used so that you can replicate it in the future. The most popular carrier oils used for aromatherapy massage oils are: sweet almond oil, cold-pressed coconut oil, grapeseed oil, jojoba oil and olive oil.

Easy DIY Diffuser Blends You Can Make Yourself

Diffusing one type of oil is good enough but what's better? Diffusing a blend of different types of oils! The following are some popular blends you can put in your diffuser:

Rejuvenating Freshness

Step into summertime freshness with a scent that hits all your limbic system senses. This blend will fill your heart with peace and love. Combine 2 drops of spearmint oil, 2 drops of grapefruit oil, and 2 drops of lemon oil and 3 drops of lavender oil in your diffuser.

Dissolve the Stench

In a household setting, stench can come from filthy sports uniform, pet odors or even the trash can. A blend of 2 drops of lemon oil, 1 drop of tea tree oil, 1 drop of lime oil and 1 drop of cilantro oil can do wonders for your home.

Is It Allergy Season Again? No Problem

Seasonal allergies can make life really miserable – whether they come in the summer or winter. With a proper blend of essential oils, the effects of your allergies will be alleviated or kept at bay. Mix 3 drops of lemon oil and 3 drops of lavender oil with 3 drops of peppermint oil in your diffuser and begin to enjoy the allergy-relieving effects of this blend.

Eliminate the Bugs

Bugs like roaches, mosquitoes, ants and houseflies can really be a nuisance around the house. Bugs typically like to hide in places like: dark spots, corners, cracks in the wall, trash cans and under the sink. An ideal diffuser blend for this is made by combining 1 drop of lemongrass oil, 1 drop of basil oil, 1 drop of thyme oil and 1 drop of eucalyptus oil.

Goodnight Princess

After a long hard day, what you are often looking forward to is a good night's rest. Essential oils can do wonders for you in your journey into slumber land. Make a blend for your diffuser by mixing 2 drops of lavender oil, 2 drops of marjoram oil and 2 drops of chamomile for pleasant night.

Chapter 7: Frequently Asked Questions

How can I use essential oils on children?

Treat essential oils like medication by keeping them out of reach of children. Some like wintergreen can be very toxic in large doses while others like melaleuca are toxic even in small doses when taken internally. When using on kids, make sure you dilute them in carrier oils or in a bath as described in the packaging. If you have to apply them topically, do it to the bottom of their feet.

Which essential oils are safe to use when pregnant?

Pregnancies are very sensitive – especially during the first trimester because your baby develops rapidly at this stage. When pregnant, always dilute your oils before using them rather than applying them directly onto your skin. Where possible, use aromatherapy instead of ingesting or topical application. Essential oils to avoid when pregnant are: Basil, Cassia, Cinnamon, Clary Sage, Lemongrass, Rosemary, Thyme, Vetiver, Wintergreen and White Fir Oils.

Is it okay to use essential oils when breastfeeding?

Some essential oils, like peppermint oil, can decrease milk supply; therefore you should minimize their usage. The packaging found in the oils will usually contain guidelines on how and when to use essential oils when breastfeeding. Generally speaking, the following oils are considered safe to use when breastfeeding (but always check with your doctor first): Ylang Ylang, Wild Orange, Sandalwood, Roman Chamomile, Patchouli, Melaleuca, Lemon, Lavender, Geranium, Grapefruit, Clary Sage and Bergamot Oils.

How much should I use?

Most essential oils are very strong; so, as a general practice, always use a little since it will go a long way. Start with just one drop and work up from there, unless you have a recipe or suggested protocol that recommends doing otherwise.

Can I use more than one blend at a time?

Yes you can. Have fun and layer the blends freely to customize the combination of your individual needs. One blend can produce different results to different people. However, some blends don't make sense in combination; for example an Invigorate blend and a sleep blend.

If I'm allergic to the plant, can I still use its essential oil?

Yes, probably. Plant allergies are to the protein of the plant: the leaf, the seed, the pollen, etc. None of that is present in the essential oil. Do your own research (and consult your doctor) and do what you feel comfortable with. You can always try the oil in an inconspicuous location to see how you respond. If you do get a rash from using oil from a plant that you are allergic to, it doesn't necessarily mean that you are allergic to the oil. It could be because you applied too much or the dilution was not enough.

Is it safe to drink essential oils internally?

Yes and no. Something that is safe for one person may not be safe for another due to things like allergies, sensitivities, or contraindicated health issues. Before deciding to take any essential oil internally, check its quality, purity, and testing. Now, if you are still confused about all this, it is best to consult with your doctor before deciding to ingest any type of essential oil.

How should I store my essential oils and blends?

Keep your oils away from direct heat and light. Store them in a dark glass bottle and in a cool and dry area. When correctly stored, your oils can stay in good condition for up to 2 years. Ideally, the best place to store your aromatherapy oils is in a dry, dark room with a temperature slightly below 68 F. Also, only buy what you are going to be using. There's no need to buy more than enough.

What precautions should I take when using essential oils?

Essential oils have multiple uses and so precautions tend to vary depending on their usage. Also, most of these precautions are described in the packaging but I'll just go ahead and summarize some of them.

- ✓ Use high quality pure oils.
- ✓ When in doubt, dilute with some carrier oil.
- ✓ It is advisable to carry out a skin test before topical application of any oil.
- ✓ Keep them out of reach of your eyes.
- ✓ In case of skin irritation, stop using the oil. If you're using it concentrated, try diluting it before using it again.

How do I tell the right blend for me?

Blend is all about what you need and what you like. If blends seem similar, try them both to see which one fits you best. Choose blends based on what they can do for you.

Bonus

Essential Oil Salad Recipes

French Cucumber Salad infused with Marjoram Essential Oil

Ingredients

- 2 toothpicks of Marjoram essential oil
- 2 tomatoes, diced
- 2 whole avocados, diced
- 2 tablespoons of olive oil
- Salt to taste
- ¾ red onion, sliced
- 1 whole cucumber, diced
- 2 tablespoons of freshly squeezed lemon juice

Method

1. In a large bowl, mix together the avocado, tomatoes, red onions and cucumber.
2. Pour olive oil into the mixture along with Marjoram essential oil
3. Add some lemon juice and salt to taste.
4. Lightly mix the ingredients once more and serve immediately.

Lemon Essential Oil Vinaigrette Salad Dressing

Ingredients

- 3 drops of Lemon Essential Oil
- Salt to taste
- 1 teaspoon of ground mustard
- 3 tablespoons of apple cider vinegar
- 2 teaspoons of pure honey
- 2 tablespoons of grated onion
- 5 tablespoons of extra virgin olive oil

Method

1. In a small bowl, combine all the ingredients together and whisk until they are well combined.
2. Pour this dressing over a variety of your favorite salads. It works well with chicken salad, tuna salad and fruit salads.

Kale Caesar Salad with Wild Orange Essential Oil Dressing

Ingredients

- A large bunch of curly kale
- A cup of sunflower seeds some of which will be used for garnish

- Sea salt to taste
- A slice of crusty bread
- 2 cloves of garlic
- 2 to 3 drops of Wild Orange Essential Oil
- ¾ cup of raw almonds, activated
- ½ teaspoon of smoked paprika
- ¼ teaspoon of chili powder
- 1¼ cups of distilled water
- 1½ teaspoons of rice malt syrup
- Parmesan cheese sprinkle

Method

1. Rinse the kale leaves and pat dry with a paper towel before cutting it up into bite size pieces and place them in a bowl.
2. Combine all the other ingredients in a blender and blend until they are nice, smooth and creamy.
3. Pour half the mixture over the kale in the bowl and mix until all of it is coated.
4. Add the remaining mixture and work it well into the kale and let it rest for 10 minutes to tenderize the leaves.

5. Plate the greens and garnish with some sunflower seeds to your satisfaction

Conclusion

You now understand that essential oils are a must have in your home. You can use them for hygiene purposes, general well-being or for mental and spiritual health. Thanks to the information provided in this book, you can start making your own custom blends and still find ways to introduce these oils to your daily diet. You have all the right tools and information to find a trustworthy and reliable essential oils dealer and are able to use these oils responsibly to benefit both yourself and your loved ones. Enjoy!

Essential Oils Guide Book

The Complete Reference Guide to Essential Oil
Remedies, Recipes, History, Uses, Safety, and How
to Choose the Best Essential Oils

Essential Oils Guide Book

The Complete Reference Guide to Essential Oil Remedies, Recipes, History, Uses, Safety, and How to Choose the Best Essential Oils

Published by CAC Publishing LLC.

ISBN 978-1-948489-88-1 paperback

ISBN 978-1-948489-87-4 eBook

Introduction

Think about the beautiful fragrance of your favorite flower. Maybe it is a rose. Maybe it's jasmine. Perhaps you have a favorite herb that you cook with, like oregano or rosemary, that evokes that wonderful aroma. All of these luscious scents come from the plant's essential oils.

Photo by Hamachidori

What Are Essential Oils?

All plants have oils that are essential to the plant's function. These oils are called "essential" because they provide essential functions and protections for the plant. These oils are extracted from the plant and bottled in a pure and highly concentrated form for all sorts of uses. The oils can be extracted from leaves and other parts of the plants by crushing or distilling to release the essential oils.

Essential oils are not really oils at all, because they don't consist of the fatty acids that make an oil an oil as we know it. They are highly concentrated plant extracts that many people consider to be the soul or life force of the plant.

How Essential Oils Help Plants

We can all take a lesson from plants and how they use essential oils and extrapolate it for our own use. Think of essential oils as a plant's active chemical compounds that serve as a built-in natural protection against the environment. The citronella plant is a great example. Have you ever used a citronella candle on your patio to ward off mosquitoes? If so, that candle is using the natural essential oil in the citronella plant to keep pests at bay.

Photo courtesy of US Department of Agriculture

Plants have oils that provide protection and healing for the plant itself. Each plant has different oils which translate to a distinctive smell for each plant. That's why roses and rosemary don't smell the same (thank goodness!) Some oils attract insects to the plant in order to pollinate it, like roses, jasmine, citrus blooms and other sweet-smelling flowers. Other oils are sharp and pungent, like citronella, telling pests to stay away.

Each oil is unique with its own microscopic building blocks called volatile aromatic compounds (VAC) that determine the oils' unique properties. These compounds are termed "volatile" because they very quickly change state from one form to another—in this case from liquid to gas. When you first open a bottle, the strong aroma comes from the oil changing into a gaseous state.

Amazingly, more than 3,000 plant VACs have been discovered by scientists worldwide. Interestingly, slightly different species of the same plant all have slightly different VACs. Oil compositions of the same species can vary depending on where the plant is grown, and climate conditions like geography, altitude, temperature and humidity.

How Essential Oils Help Humans

Essential oils work for plants, so why wouldn't they work for humans? The essential oil VAC building blocks are molecules small enough to penetrate your cells. Essential oils differ from other oils like fatty vegetable oils which are larger molecules too large to penetrate cells. Therefore, they can be used for cooking, but not for therapeutic health benefit.

All of the protective, healing qualities that the plants possess in their stems, bark, roots, leaves and flowers have been harnessed and bottled into the essential oils we humans use today.

The Market For Essential Oils

The harnessing and bottling market is a huge global market. Indeed, a new report by Grand View Research shows that the global market for essential oils will reach nearly $14 billion in just a few years, by 2024. Essential oils have exploded onto the scene as more and more people seek natural remedies and organic products. Today, people all over the world use essential oils for a wide range of physical and emotional applications. Oils are used as single oils or can be mixed with other oils to create powerful and complex essential oil blends.

History of Essential Oils

In today's modern world, we have so many synthetic products. More and more, people are shying away from synthetics and opting for more natural products like the essential oils. Ancient people didn't have synthetics and had to naturally rely on botanicals. The modern essential oil market represents the evolution of thousands of years of essential oils use. Indeed, many modern pharmaceuticals are derived from plants. Let's explore the history, shall we?

The ancient world was heavily intermingled with the plant world. They used plant extracts for religion, medicine, food preparation and beauty.

Egypt

The earliest written and recorded uses of essential oils were in Egypt, where plant life flourished thanks to the very fertile Nile River valley. Historical records show that Egypt had an abundance of food and a booming agricultural industry. The Egyptian civilization was progressive in many ways, including urban planning, government, and most of all medicine.

Historians reference the 1500 B.C. Ebers Papyrus as one of the earliest known medical texts from Egypt. It is believed to have been a copy from earlier texts dating back to 3000 B.C. The scroll contains rituals for medical ceremonies, recipes, and uses of botanicals for all kinds of things, including mummification.

Of course, Egypt wrote the book (literally) on how to mummify bodies in preparation for burial, and this early text references use of juniper, cedar and cinnamon oils in preparing the bodies.

Egyptians used oils not just for mummification, but also in many aspects of everyday life, in many religious ceremonies and herbal remedies for medical purposes. The Egyptian culture had a focus on beauty, and many plant oils were used to concoct beauty treatments. The famous Egyptian queen Cleopatra was given a wonderful gift by her love Marc Antony—he gave her a spa near the Dead Sea. Clearly Antony is a man after every girl's heart, and Cleopatra regularly used the spa's natural resources like salt, clay, and essential oils to maintain her legendary beauty.

Egypt's ruling pharaoh families wore expensive perfumes made from essential oils, and temple priests used many oils for spiritual ceremonies. These priests also doubled as doctors, so they used many oils to prepare medicines and ointments.

Amazingly, archaeologists have discovered ancient pictorial hieroglyphics on Egyptian temple walls that show essential oils being extracted and used. Plants and their oils were revered in the Egyptian culture. When scientists found King Tutankhamen's tomb in 1922, they discovered over 50 alabaster jars thought to hold essential oils, left there for the pharaoh to use in the afterlife.

Although historians largely give credit to Egypt as the first culture to widely use essential oils, it turns out that ancient China and India were also using these oils around the same time period.

China

In China, plants have been an integral part of medicine for centuries, and continue to be today. The 2700 B.C. text known as Shennong's Herbal is the oldest known Chinese text. It contains details on how the ancient Chinese healers used nearly 400 medicinal plants. Shennong is regarded as the father of Chinese herbal medicine; he was also a ruler who taught the people agriculture. Shennong used himself as a guinea pig and ingested hundreds of herbs and plants to test their effects. He is largely credited as being the discoverer of tea and the inventor of acupuncture. Like Shennong, Huangdi, also called the Yellow Emperor, wrote a book on medicine which detailed the important use of essential oils. Amazingly, Huangdi's book is still used by Chinese medicine practitioners to this day. Indeed, China is the largest producer of essential oils in the world today.

India

Like in China, ancient India used essential oils as a core part of their Ayurvedic practices. Still used today, Ayurvedic practice is a naturopathic approach to healing that combines practical elements of medicine with spiritual and philosophical beliefs.

Although historians cannot accurately pinpoint a beginning, Ayurvedic medicine is thought to have been practiced for at least 5,000 years. Indeed it is still widely practiced in India, as well as other parts of the world, even today.

One of the principle Ayurvedic practices is aromatherapy and massage. Indian literature, as far back as 2000 B.C., discusses doctors' use of oils like cinnamon, ginger and sandalwood with massage to ease patient symptoms.

The term "Ayurveda" means "life knowledge", and the Indian sacred text known as the Vedas mentions more than 700 different plants and herbs used for religious and medical purposes. For example, basil is considered a sacred plant of India. It is believed to bestow the properties of energy, love and devotion, and also believed to have the power to open one's heart and mind. Basil is widely accepted in India and used to strengthen compassion, faith and clarity of thought.

Ayurvedic principles have worldwide influence in modern times, thanks to practitioners like Deepak Chopra and other people across the globe who have established training institutions.

Greeks

The ancient Greeks and Romans derived much of their knowledge from the Egyptians, including use of essential oils. The Greek father of modern medicine, Hippocrates, kept records of medicinal uses for over 300 plants. He still influences medicine today as doctors still take the Hippocratic oath in his name. Hippocrates often prescribed hot baths with aromatic oils added to the water and massage with essential oils.

During Hippocrates lifetime, a plague hit Athens, and he fumigated the city with essential oils to keep the pestilence from spreading. Today, we know that plague is caused by an infectious bacteria, and we also know that oils, like oregano, have antibacterial properties. Although Hippocrates did not have our modern knowledge, he was obviously on the right track. He always prescribed all kinds of essential oil treatments for wounded soldiers on the battlefields.

Hippocrates' colleague Theophrastus talked about the "perfumes", meaning essential oils with medicinal properties because of the effects they had on various ailments. He talked of plasters and poultices being used to treat abscesses and tumors as well as internal injuries. Interestingly, the Greeks had already figured out that if these oils are applied externally to the skin, they seep in to repair internal tissues. Indeed, oils are widely used today for this very purpose.

Romans

Like the Greeks, ancient Romans were influenced by Egyptians and the Greeks, particularly in the area of health care. More than any culture before them, Romans used essential oils voluminously. They ate them, they drank them, they bathed in them, they breathed them in, and they had massages using them. The oils were a part of daily life. In particular, the Romans were bath fanatics and known to bathe up to several times a day in waters laced with essential oils. They used oils for hair and body care, and scented their beds with oils like lavender, a practice still widely done today. Romans had master perfumers, who used the most exotic oils to create amazing blends.

Greek physician Dioscorides was employed as an army doctor in Rome, and he wrote a multi-volume book on herbal medicine in 1 A.D. In the book were

600 remedies, many which are still used today. He wrote about juniper berry as a diuretic, marjoram as a sedative, and cypress for treating diarrhea.

Essential oils are even mentioned in the Christian Bible. Shortly after Christ's birth, the three wise men brought gifts of frankincense and myrrh, two of the oldest essential oils. The Bible has dozens of references to medicinal plants, and mentions at least 12 essential oils, like cinnamon and cedarwood. In the story of Moses's Exodus, the Bible mentions a holy anointing oil containing cassia, clove and olive oils.

Middle Ages – Europe

In the Middle Ages, essential oil use experienced a temporary setback when the Catholic Church denounced many of Hippocrates' teachings, like bathing for healing. Despite the Pope's ruling, many monks kept using plant medicine as cures in their villages, and by the 1600s, herbal medicine was once again widely used. By the 1800s, most of Europe's pharmacies, such as in England, Germany and France, were using and prescribing essential oils for a variety of illnesses.

In France, large flower growers were also using the oils as a commercial business by supplying them to the perfume houses which the French are still known for today. One day, scientists took notice that men who worked at the flower growers were generally healthy, even though disease like tuberculosis were sweeping the rest of France. The curiosity of these early researchers led to the first known laboratory test of anti-bacterial properties of the oils in 1887.

Later, in 1910, a scientific discovery occurred by accident, as so many often do. French chemist Rene-Maurice Gattefosse suffered severe burns to his hands and arms as a result of a laboratory explosion. His hands quickly showed signs of severe blistering so he used the only remedy he had and dipped his hands into a large container of lavender oil. Gattefosse was astonished that one dip stopped the burning.

Gattefosse was a chemist, but wasn't interested in medicine until his personal experience changed his path. He soon began investigating how oils could be used to treat World War I soldiers. Gattefosse is famous for creating the term "aromatherapie". Several decades later, Parisian medical doctor Jean Valnet, followed in Gattefosse's footsteps in another moment of serendipity. He ran out of antibiotics during the Indochina War in the 1950s. Remembering Gattefosse's story, he began using essential oils as antiseptics. Since he was stationed in China, the oils were in ready supply. Valnet credited the oils for saving many soldiers. After the war, he continued his research and even published an authoritative text entitled The Practice of Aromatherapy in 1964. The book is still widely recognized today as the basis for the modern global essential oil movement.

Exhibit in the Tekniska Museet, Stockholm, Sweden

Twenty years later, more French scientists, Daniel Pénoël and Pierre Franchomme, provided clinical uses for over 270 essential oils and published their book L'aromatherapie Exactement in 1990, still used today as the primary reference book for medical benefits of essential oils.

Health Benefits of Essential Oils

Clearly, ancient cultures and modern-day scientists were on to something. What they knew from observation, modern scientists know from research and detailed knowledge of how cells function. Today, we know the exact mechanisms of how essential oils work.

Antibacterial

Scientists have turned to essential oils as an alternative to antibiotics, which bacteria are increasingly becoming resistant to. "The loss of antibiotics due to antimicrobial resistance is potentially one of the most important challenges the medical and animal-health communities will face in the 21st century," says Dr. Cyril Gay, the senior national program leader at the United States Department of Agriculture (USDA).

Some estimates predict that these drug-resistant bacteria will cause more than 10 million deaths in the next 30 years, by 2050.

Livestock consume antibiotics, and then the meat is consumed by humans. The out-of-control use in agriculture has led to the creation of superbugs with dire consequences to humans. The large majority of antibiotics used on livestock are also used to treat human diseases, and that is why the consequences are so dire. The USDA has turned to essential oils research as a potential antibiotic alternative, and some of it has been very promising. An October 2014 study showed that oregano oil fed to chickens greatly reduced the occurrence of a common poultry infection called ascites.

In another study, a feed meal made of oregano, cinnamon and chili peppers suppressed a common intestinal infection and even resulted in the chickens gaining more weight. Another team of researchers used a similar concoction of turmeric, chili pepper, and shiitake mushrooms. The USDA is currently conducting a multi-year study examining the use of several essential oils like citrus oils as antibiotic alternatives.

The USDA and other researchers have compared antibiotics with essential oil use and have found them to be comparable. In one example, rosemary and oregano oils had similar results to the common poultry antibiotic avilamycin. At the University of Georgia, a blend of oils was effective at stopping the spread of salmonella. There is strong evidence that these essential oils are very effective against the intestinal bacteria that often affect livestock.

Human research has shown similar promising results, although the studies are rare and tend to be smaller scale studies. American researchers have studied tea tree oil and its effect on staph infections; wounds treated with the oil healed faster, and lemongrass oil reduced the antibiotic resistant dangerous form of staph called MRSA.

Many scientific labs around the globe are testing all kinds of combinations of essential oils, and consistently, research shows that these oils can fight numerous pathogens, regular and antibiotic-resistant. Even when antibiotics are given, using oils can reduce the amount of drugs a person must take. Basil oil and rosemary oil slowed the growth of 60 strains of *E. coli* typically found in hospital settings.

The oils work to weaken the bacterial cell wall, which damages the cell to let antibiotics in to work their magic.

Johns Hopkins' Dr. Nicole M. Parrish says an alternative is sorely needed. She often encounters patients where no antibiotic is effective, a situation which makes her feel helpless as a physician. Parrish says that essential oils are some of the most potent antimicrobial fighters on the planet, and it is crucial to further that understanding to bring about a new class of drugs.

Here are some of the top antibacterial essential oils.

- Cinnamon oil has been shown to be an effective antibacterial agent. In a dental study, it was effective against a type of common bacteria *E. faecalis* that people are susceptible to after having a root canal. The oil eliminated the bacteria altogether by eradicating its biofilm. The oil has also been used agriculturally to fight bacteria in strawberry plants.

- <u>Thyme</u> is another effective antimicrobial shown to be effective against salmonella commonly found in milk of dairy cattle.

- <u>Oregano</u> has long been used to fight respiratory bacterial infections and is now being used to fight antibiotic resistant infections. Oregano studies have shown the oil to be very effective against certain drug-resistant bacterial strains by disruption of the bacterial cell structure and function.

- <u>Tea tree oil</u> has long been used as a topical ointment for skin infections. New research shows that tea tree oil was very effective against staphylococcus and *E. coli*. After the oil was applied, it had an immediate effect on these bacteria, and continued to whittle away for 24 hours.

Antifungal

Fungal infections are very hard to kill. That's because a fungus is similar to human cells. Genes are similar and so are cellular processes, so when you try to kill a fungus, it often ends up impacting the human in a very detrimental way. While there are many antibiotics on the market today to kill bacteria, which are relatively easy to kill, there are only three classes of antifungal drugs. Furthermore, fungi are becoming readily resistant to these drugs.

The only real difference between a human cell and a fungal cell is that the fungus has something called chitin in its cell wall; humans do not. Other organisms also have chitin—organisms like nematodes and protozoa. Most organisms that have chitin end up being pathogens to other species like humans. Chitin is a protein, and under normal circumstances, the human immune system recognizes chitin as a foreign invader and the body deals with it. Cells in the lungs and gastrointestinal tract have chitin receptors to sense an invasion and activate the immune system. Skin does as well. However, sometimes a person's immune response is not functioning properly, so the body cannot clear itself of the chitin. A great example is when a person is allergic to dust mites, which have chitin in their exoskeletons. The person's lungs do not properly detect the mites' chitin, and an allergy develops.

For this reason, fungal infections are opportunistic, often affecting people with other diseases and compromised immune systems. Chemicals have been shown to be largely ineffective for killing fungi, but essential oils are very promising in fighting these invaders. Here's how they accomplish that.

Fungi form biofilms that help them remain hardy in the host environment. These biofilms help them strongly attach to healthy human cells, and the biofilm also provides an extra support matrix for the cell wall. Scientists who have studied biofilms show that they provide a protective shield against the human environment, like a layer of extra protection, making them even harder to eradicate. In a medical setting, when a fungus forms its biofilm, it helps the fungus adhere to urinary catheters and other medical apparatus. Once they're on the equipment, they can easily gain access to the bloodstream or urinary organs. Yeast is such a fungus, explaining why so many people in the hospital also develop secondary yeast infections. Once the fungi develop the biofilm, they become even more resistant to antifungal drugs. Research on biofilms is relatively new and there are still many things that scientists don't know about how they work, but they do know that once fungi cells are inside a biofilm, these cells actually communicate with each other for group survival. It's a little creepy, but it shows how hardy the fungi truly are. As the biofilm gains strength, it begins resisting the human body's natural defenses, which over time become less and less effective against the fungus.

Essential oils show promise because they break down the fortress wall of a biofilm. Some drugs do this too, but then they don't kill the fungi inside the biofilm. Essential oils do both. For example, tea tree oil (melaleuca) is very effective against the yeast species Candida albicans; it not only bores through the biofilm, it keeps new fungal cells from forming. Other oils like cinnamon appear to keep the biofilm from forming in the first place. In other trials of the *Mentha suaveolens* plant which is native to Morocco, the essential oil of the plant was found to shut down the metabolic factory of the fungus cells by about 80 percent, rendering them virtually inactive and greatly impaired. Citronella oil is another well-known antifungal oil.

Essential oils are also effective in treating a "super biofilm" called a polymicrobial biofilms, formed by a mixture of bacteria and fungi. These biofilms often occur in patients with chronic infections, and oils like clove, eucalyptus and peppermint have proven effective.

In some trials, eucalyptus has performed better than the common antifungal drug fluconazole. Lemongrass essential oil seems to deform and shrink fungus cells.

Anise oil was found to be very effective against a particular type of filamentous fungus, and other oils are found to alter structures and functions inside the fungal cells.

Many plants have two oils that work synergistically together to help or protect the plant, and researchers have found that they continue to work that way in humans. For example, oregano and thyme oil by themselves are great antifungal agents. Researchers have determined that they're even more effective when they work together. They've isolated the compounds carvacrol and thymol in each oil, and when put together cause much more damage to the cell membrane, block toxin production from the fungal cells, and can even cause death of the fungus.

Unfortunately, more and more people are getting fungal infections. The main culprit is *candida* yeast because people are eating more sugar and processed foods that serve as a breeding ground for *candida*. Furthermore, antibiotic overuse creates more fungal infections as they become drug resistant just like bacteria do.

Fungal infections are the cause of so many pesky ailments like toenail fungus, jock itch, vaginal infections and body odor.

However, these essential oils can come to your rescue.

- Lavender has been compared to the antifungal drug clotrimazole for vaginal yeast infections, and researchers found that after 48 hours, there was no difference between the two. This means that given sufficient time, lavender can be effective against these infections.

- Thyme is effective against several different strains of gut bacteria and fungi.

- Peppermint is a well-known oil for stomach upset and it was recently tested against 12 fungal strains and was effective on 11 of them.

- Geranium has been used for centuries to promote healthy skin. It was also an oil that was able to stop or slow the growth of 12 fungal strains tested.

- Bitter almond must be used with extreme caution in humans, but it has been shown to be very effective for agricultural use against 19 common fungal strains that affect crops. It shows promise as a natural pesticide.

- Black pepper is high in antioxidants. Scientists have isolated the chemical compounds in the oil of the pepper plant Piper divaricatum and found strong antifungal agents that are effective even when administered in very low doses.

- Cinnamon has been used since ancient times as an antiviral and antiparasitic agent, but now that scientists have isolated its compounds, it is also shown to be an antifungal and antimicrobial.

- Citronella is well known as a mosquito and insect repellent, but it is also very effective against respiratory infections and was recently found to be effective against seven separate fungal strains.

- Clove helps in gum disease and treats acne, but it is also very effective against candida strains. Clove practically wipes candida out!

- Eucalyptus has helped asthma and pneumonia sufferers for years. The oil is commonly found in products to treat the common cold. The oil is also a very effective antifungal.

Antiviral

Hundreds of published studies show essential oil effectiveness against viruses. Oils are "fat friendly" and since our cell membranes are lined with fats, the oils easily pass through.

Viruses wreak so much havoc in the human body because they have a tough outer shell called a capsid that protects the virus once it enters the human host.

This is why influenza, called an enveloped virus, affects so many people each year. Furthermore, viruses use their own cell walls to fuse with healthy human cell walls in a kind of cellular takeover of the healthy cell. Once they do that, the virus easily replicates.

Oils like lavender and melissa have been shown to inactivate that tough outer coating. The oils either break down the virus cell wall so that it can't fuse to a human cell, or the oils prevent the virus from replicating.

Interestingly, scientists have isolated the active compounds in the oils and have tested that isolated compound as well as the whole oil complex against the virus. For example, tea tree oil was tested against its active compound called terpinen-4-ol. Amazingly, for tea tree as well as several other oils studied in a similar fashion, the whole oil worked ten times better than the isolated compound. Although more research is required, scientists think this is due to the synergistic effects of the oil's compounds—two substances that work together and are better than each part used separately.

Immune oil blends are even more effective because they combine several essential oils to fight the virus on all fronts.

Here are a few of the best antiviral oils:

- Peppermint Oil can do a real number on viruses, particularly the herpes virus that causes cold sores. It can also treat symptoms of the virus that causes the common cold— symptoms like sore throat and congestion.

- Thyme Oil kills viruses while at the same time relieving symptoms. It is particularly effective in respiratory infections, as well as herpes virus. It is often used in an immune blend along with cinnamon and clove.

- Rosemary is best known for cooking, but it is very effective against influenza virus, the common cold and herpes viruses.

- Lavender oil is calming but it is also a powerful antiviral agent used to treat the common cold, flu and cold sores.

- Pine oil is a lesser known essential oil that has been tested against multiple strains of the herpes virus with great results. The oil has high levels of antiviral activity, even against drug-resistant viruses.

- Eucalyptus oil is commonly found in over the counter cold remedies, but it is also a powerful antifungal. It works very well on herpes virus cold sores and blisters.

How Do Essential Oils Work?

The chemistry of these essential oils holds the key to how they work. Basically, the oils consist of oxygenated molecules and hydrocarbons that give the oils their effective properties.

Terpenes make up the main hydrocarbon in essential oils. Terpenes are what give the oils their strong aromas. They are present in varying amounts, depending on the oil. For example, the terpene limonene is present in nearly 100 percent concentrations in citrus oils like lemon, wild orange, bergamot and grapefruit. Citronella's terpenes protect it from insects. Every plant has terpenes.

Terpenes are what make a rose smell like a rose and a blueberry smell like a blueberry. Terpenes are secreted by the plant to be attractive to insects for pollination, sticky to trap insects, or pungent to ward off insects. Although terpenes are similar in plant species, they can vary slightly in plants grown in different regions and climates.

In humans, terpenes are protective to the cells. They help promote cell growth and have great antioxidant qualities. When the oil is absorbed through the skin, it is the terpenes that bind to your cell or brain receptors to create the effects that oil is known for.

Terpenes can be subdivided into smaller groups. Monoterpenes help the cell from building up toxins, and they help support the DNA in every cell. Citrus oils as well as oils like pine, cedar and balsam are high in monoterpenes.

Sesquiterpenes are another subgroup. These are the largest group of terpenes, and they give the oils their thickness. Cells have memory, and sesquiterpenes help to filter out bad information from cellular memory. Oils like myrrh, sandalwood and cedarwood have high levels of sesquiterpenes.

Phenolics are another important compound found in essential oils. They function as "housekeepers" to make sure receptor sites on cells are clean and able to bind to important chemicals. They work with sesquiterpenes by cleaning the receptor first, which allows the sesquiterpenes to then bind to the cell to do their work. Phenolics also have antioxidant properties. Tea tree, wintergreen and clove oils are high in phenolics.

Certain essential oils are high in alcohols, which give the cell its oxidation resistance. They also help the cell to function normally. Geranium and rosewood oils are high in alcohols.

Are Essential Oils Safe?

Most essential oils are safe when used properly. Anytime you're introduced to something new, it's a good idea to proceed conservatively, and the same is true with oils.

Essential oils are classified as GRAS or Generally Recognized As Safe by the U.S. Food and Drugs

Administration (FDA). Very few people have adverse side effects when these oils are properly used. There are several factors to keep in mind.

Dosage

Just as with medication, dosage is a very important part of essential oil safety. Using oil in high doses can do harm; for example, they can cause a skin reaction if used topically and incorrectly.

Dose is important to follow regardless of how you're using the oil, whether aromatically, topically, or internally.

Remember that an essential oil dose will always depend on the age, size, health status, and personal skin sensitivity of the individual. If you have specific concerns about your skin, it is always a good idea to consult with your physician before using essential oils topically.

Dose will vary depending on your health status, age and weight. When using an essential oil for the first time, always start with the lowest possible dose, around one or two drops, see how your body reacts to the small dose, then increase over time according to package directions.

It is important to always remember that oils are very concentrated and thus very potent. So, it is better to use a few small doses periodically throughout the day instead of using or taking a single large dose.

Most aromatherapy oil-based blends of more than one oil are between one and five percent dilutions, so they don't pose a safety risk.

Application Methods

Some oils can be used aromatically, topically and ingested, while others have a specific single application. Always follow directions. Some oils are safe topically, but cause issues when inhaled, and vice versa.

Before you use an oil, make sure you know its recommended application method, as well as the concentration and dosage. Never ingest oils without professional guidance.

Since most essential oils cannot be applied directly to the skin without dilution, don't forget to use your carrier oil.

Sensitivity

All people are different—with different chemical compositions, health status and makeups. Therefore, it is possible for any oil to cause sensitivity. Children are more likely to have a sensitivity response so extra safety precautions should be taken. Oils are generally not a good idea for children under age seven.

You can apply an oil topically as a form of sensitivity test when first using the oil. Use one drop with a carrier oil and see how your skin reacts. Check the test area every hour.

Some oils can slightly change composition if exposed to the sun or UV light, because their compounds are photosensitive. Citrus oils, in particular, have this issue, but oil manufacturers will usually post it on the label. The light sensitivity can change the oil and you might become more sun-sensitive as a result. The potency of oil can affect children. Some oils should be avoided altogether, while others should only be used in a highly diluted form and under the guidance of a knowledgeable professional. For example, wintergreen and birch should never be used on children due to the high concentrations of methyl salicylate.

Purity

Always make sure to use pure essential oils. There are some imposters on the market that contain alterations like addition of synthetic chemicals or dilutions with vegetable oil. The label should indicate purity. Note that some expensive oils like rose oil (at $100 a teaspoon) are sometimes sold in diluted form, but it will be advertised on the label.

Just know that oils that are not pure have an increased likelihood of creating an adverse response, so it is very important to only buy pure and genuine essential oils.

Drug Interactions

Not much research has been done on interactions of essential oils with standard pharmaceutical drugs, but it does make sense that it could happen, due to the complex chemical nature of the oils.

It's always important, if you're on prescription medications, to talk over use of any new product with your doctor. More research is being done every day, like a study showing that peppermint and eucalyptus oils increase the skin absorption of the anti-cancer drug called 5-fluorouracil.

Certain oils are known to interact with blood thinner medications, like clary sage, cypress, eucalyptus, ginger, rosemary, sage and thyme.

Toxicity

Rarely does a toxic event occur with appropriate use of essential oils. Toxicity is typically due to misuse or accidental ingestion of an oil, particularly by children.

There are some oils that have been banned by The International Fragrance Association which monitors the industry. They've banned certain essential oils because they have been found to be toxic when ingested or applied topically: cade oil crude, costus root, elecampane, fig leaf absolute, horseradish, nightshade, pennyroyal, rue, sassafras, savin, southernwood, stinging nettle, stryax gum, tea absolute, wormseed and wormwood.

How Are Essential Oils Produced?

Oils must be extracted from the plant parts and bottled effectively as a product. There are several methods for producing and extracting essential oils.

Distillation

Steam distillation is a common method for extracting essential oils from plants. The plant parts are put onto a grid and boiling water is placed underneath. As the steam rises, the oils are literally pulled out of the plant. The steam and the oil rise together and it is captured in a jar-like container and drained using tubing. The oil/water mixture is rapidly cooled and since water and oils don't mix, the two are separated and the oil is collected. Depending on the oil, the remaining water can sometimes contain some of the aromatic compounds of the plant. This water by-product is called a hydrosol and is very fragrant and used in cosmetic products.

Expression

Expression is the most direct way to extract an essential oil. This method involves pressing the oil-containing plant parts—leaves, seeds, flowers, skins—

in a process very similar to how olive oil is made. For example, expression is used on citrus rinds to press the oil out of the skins.

Carbon Dioxide

Extraction of oils using carbon dioxide (CO_2) is a relatively new and interesting process that has been around for approximately 10 years. It is a very expensive process, but results in a very high quality oil. Compressed CO_2 is used in a high pressure, low temperature process to extract the oil from botanicals.

Solvents

While chemical solvents can be used to extract oils from the plants, most producers prefer not to use this method out of concern that trace elements of the chemicals will be left behind. In this method, the plant is completely dissolved in solvents like benzene or methylene. Then the solvent is removed via evaporation using a vacuum or centrifuge device to pull the solvent from the essential oil. The oil product that results is called an "absolute". This process is very expensive, and usually reserved for expensive oils which can't be distilled (rose, vanilla, jasmine).

Enfleurage

Enfleurage is a very old traditional method only used in France today because it requires a high skill level and is complicated and very expensive. Flower blossoms are placed in warm fat that absorbs the oil out of the flowers. The French used to use lard or animal fat but now use vegetable fats in the process. The flowers are then removed and the process is repeated several times. Once enough oil is in the fats, the two are separated to leave just the essential oil product.

How To Use Essential Oils

Essential oils can be used in many versatile ways: aromatic, topical and even by internal ingestion. Each oil has an ideal use or can perhaps be used in all these ways. As scientists conduct more research, they're developing a greater understanding of application methods specific to each oil.

Oils have amazing physical and emotional wellness applications. You can use single oils, or a complex blend of oils specially formulated for specific health applications, such as mood enhancing or respiratory. Let's explore some of the ways oils can be used.

Aromatic

Because they are volatile, and thus change state from solid to gas quickly, essential oils rapidly disperse through the air, so they're excellent for aromatherapy applications.

One of the most popular uses for essential oils is aromatherapy for emotional wellness. The receptors in our noses (olfactory receptors) quickly absorb the oil's scent. The olfactory nerve sends that signal to the limbic system, a part of the brain responsible for emotions, memory and behavior. In this process, hormones are released in your body. Think back to the last time you smelled roses; perhaps it evoked a memory of the person who brought you the bouquet, or a memory of playing in your grandmother's rose garden as a child. These are examples of your limbic system at work.

Some essential oils like citrus oils (grapefruit, orange, lemon or bergamot) are uplifting and invigorating, as are oils like peppermint and rosemary. Other oils like lavender and chamomile are calming. You may have had chamomile tea to calm yourself before bedtime; using chamomile oil is the same concept. The oils stimulate physical and emotional responses because the oils affect your mood and emotions. You'll likely be drawn to your favorite aromas instinctively.

The easiest way to do aromatherapy is to put a few drops of oil in your hands, rub them together, cup your hands over your nose and inhale the delicious aroma.

Diffusers

As this is not always practical, many people use a device called a diffuser. Using a diffuser is one of the easiest ways to use oils aromatically.

Terra cotta: There are some inexpensive diffuser options, like terra cotta jars or discs, a dish and candle or an electric plug-in scent pad. Terra-cotta is the burnt orange pottery you think of when you think of a regular flower pot.

The ceramic material is porous, so using a terra cotta container filled with oil means the oil will seep through the walls and infuse the air with scent. You can also buy sticks with terra cotta tops. Get a small glass jar and fill with oil. The oil will seep up the wooden sticks into the terra cotta tops and fill the air with aroma.

Some people even wear terra cotta pendants like a necklace; the back is glazed to prevent oil from getting on your skin or clothing. Larger terra cotta disks are available and work the same as the pendant. Think of it as a coaster you can infuse with oil! The back is glazed to prevent oil from leaking onto your furniture.

A terra cotta diffuser is a great way to get the oil aroma without using any powered device—just know that the oils disperse continuously. In short, there's no off switch. You can always put the disc in a plastic bag if you don't want the aroma at certain times.

A terra cotta diffuser is best used with the same oil. Switch to another oil only after the first oil is completely evaporated. Otherwise the oils will mix and may produce an unpleasant smell.

Candle diffuser: A candle diffuser is also a simple method of aromatherapy. A dish containing water and a few drops of oil sits on top of a candle, which provides the heat to diffuse the oil. Since essential oils don't dissolve in water, this is an effective way to scent a room. The candle is enough to heat but not boil the water, so the oils evaporate. Always use water and not oil directly, and keep an eye on the water as it evaporates so that you are not heating an empty dish. These oils are called volatile for a reason; they will quickly burn onto the surface of the dish, likely ruining your diffuser and creating a burnt aroma—not what you were going for at all! Just know that essential oils should never be directly burned. This is very dangerous, and direct burning changes the chemical structure of the oil so that it is no longer affected.

You can reuse a candle diffuser; just make sure you've thoroughly washed the dish before you use a different oil. If oils have ever burned onto the dish and can't be easily cleaned, you might not be able to reuse the dish. Certainly, over time, the dish will wear out and you'll have to buy a new dish to go with the candle diffuser. Within time, the dish, but not the whole diffuser, will need to be replaced.

As with all candles, safety is important. Never leave a candle diffuser unattended and never use overnight due to fire risk. Many people use essential oils at night as a sleep remedy, but a candle diffuser is not a good option for this use.

Electric Diffusers: An electric diffuser is a good option for anytime and anywhere you want to use oils. They don't involve an open flame and are much safer. However, they do require power: battery, plug in or USB. Some diffusers come with all three options. This is the best option for overnight use because it does not require constant monitoring.

The best way to use oils for inhalation is to purchase an essential oils diffuser. Water is placed in the device along with a few drops of a single oil or more than one oil to create an oil blend. The diffuser creates a fine mist vapor. It's a great way to scent a room.

Electric diffusers use cool water in a chamber. You add a few drops of oil to the water and the device makes a cool mist that fills the room. There are many inexpensive options on the market. Some are battery-powered, so they're transportable to use anywhere, and some have USB cables to run off your computer or even in your car. And speaking of your car, there are even smaller options that plug into a USB or lighter outlet. Many diffusers have an automatic shutoff option, so when the device runs out of water, the motor shuts off so as to not burn out the unit.

This type of diffuser can give you a wider disbursement of aroma because the vapor mist more easily fills the room. Most diffusers require about a cup of water with about 5 drops of oil directly added to the water. You can add different oils, such as orange, lemon and grapefruit for a citrus powerhouse!

Electric diffusers are generally safe. They release small amounts of vapor into the air and are very unlikely to cause the concentration of any essential oil to rise to unsafe levels. If the fragrance is too intense, raise a window to ventilate the room.

Diffusers should generally be used for about 30 minutes at a time, and try to avoid leaving your diffuser plugged in overnight. You can purchase a diffuser that has an automatic shutoff in case you forget to turn it off.

Because they are flammable, keep all oils and diffusers away from open flames. Don't overfill your diffuser, and never add carrier oils as it will gunk up the mechanism. Because diffusers use water, you're not required to add a carrier oil.

To keep your diffuser working properly, periodically wash it with soap and warm water. If stagnant water is left sitting, mold can grow, particularly in humid environments, and you certainly don't want to be misting mold into your home.

On a related note, essential oils should never be added to a humidifier, which are not made for this purpose.

Other Aromatherapy Methods

Aromatherapy is certainly not a new concept. It's been practiced for thousands of years. If you don't have a diffuser readily available, there are lots of other ways you can enjoy aromatherapy.

Dry evaporation: place oil on a cotton ball and allow it to evaporate into the air. Some people even put oil-infused cotton balls inside their car air vents for a fresh interior.

Steam: Add drops of essential oil to a steaming bowl of water. This can serve as a mini-facial spa treatment if you let the steam open your pores. Or you can place a towel over the bowl, put your head under it, and inhale the vapors. Please realize this is a very intense, direct way to inhale oils so one or two drops is enough. Lots of people use a steam containing eucalyptus essential oil to relieve nasal congestion.

Personal inhaler: You can purchase either a plastic inhaler or aluminum inhaler. Both have a wick and you can add essential oil to it, then cap for later use. Anytime you need a boost, uncap and waft under your nose. Most inhalers last a few months; just refill with oil when you feel it's lost its effectiveness.

Smelling salts: Along the same lines as the personal inhaler, you can make your own smelling salts. Just use 1 tablespoon of rock salt with 10 drops of your favorite oil. Store the mixture in a tightly-sealed container and use whenever you need a boost of clear thought.

Spray: Purchase a small sprayer bottle, add water and drops of essential oil, shake, and you have just made your own air freshener. Make sure the bottle is set for a fine mist spray. Lots of people spray the air or spray fabric furniture or rugs to freshen them up. You can also do it for curtains and comforters, or even use as a disinfecting spray by choosing an antibacterial oil to spray on kitchen counters, yoga mats, pet areas and other places where germs like to hide.

Add oil to other products: Add oil to your laundry detergent or dryer sheets for an added boost. You can even add oils to a cool light bulb (emphasis on cool). As the bulb heats, the aroma disperses. Or, ceramic round donut-shaped diffuser rings are specifically made for this purpose. You put the oil on the ring and slip the ceramic over the light bulb.

Perfume: many believers in essential oil even make their own perfume. Mix 25 drops of oil with an ounce of either perfume alcohol or denatured alcohol. Depending on the oil you choose, you might also need a carrier oil which is discussed below. Sweet almond oil or coconut oil are good choices for perfume carrier oils.

Best Aromatherapy Oils

Relaxation: for relaxation, lavender is frequently used, as is chamomile. Use this in the evening to calm your busy mind before sleep.

Sleep: Marjoram oil is another wonderful sleep-inducing oil.

Congestion: eucalyptus, peppermint or juniper are great for stuffy noses. There are even respiratory blend oils you can buy that are already mixed for you.

Skin: Tea tree oil in a steam facial can work wonders for skin problems.

Energy: Lots of people swear by citrus oils to get them up and going for the day. These oils are great mood boosters.

Cleaner: for a fresh clean scent all around your house, use lemon.

Holidays: spray pine, peppermint or clove oil for the holiday spirit.

Is Aromatherapy Safe?

Now that you know about different diffuser types, aromatherapy methods and oils, you might be wondering if it is safe to inhale essential oils. Indirect methods are very safe, but direct inhalation right out of the bottle, or by the steam or personal inhaler method warrant a few cautions.

First, these direct methods are not recommended for pregnant women or children under age 7. If you're steaming under a towel, either close your eyes or wear protective gear like swim goggles to protect your eyes. Some oils are very potent.

It is also recommended that you not use eucalyptus oil if you have asthma. Instead, pine oil is a safer substitute. Always consult your doctor.

Inhalation of oils remains a very low risk level to most people. The concentration of oil in the room is unlikely to ever get to a dangerous level. If you have prolonged exposure to highly oil-concentrated vapor—exposure of more than an hour—you might feel sluggish or have headaches, dizziness or nausea.

Topical

Topical application of essential oils is fast, simple, and effective. Used topically, oils are soothing in massage and excellent for the skin. With topical application, you can target specific areas of your body.

Molecules in the oil penetrate the skin and seep into tissues, muscles and joints. They easily penetrate the skin because they're lipid soluble, and once through, they stay in the local area to provide their benefits. As you might imagine, topical application is very effective.

Oils can calm, moisturize, reduce inflammation and help your cells eliminate waste products.

Oils are easily absorbed, but you can increase absorption by lightly massaging the area to stimulate blood flow.

Carrier Oils

You can also use an oil called a carrier oil to not only increase absorption but to help dilute stronger oils that may cause skin irritation when applied topically.

Carrier oils can also help to slow the evaporation rate of the oil on your skin.

Oils like basil, oregano and tea tree are very strong, and applied alone, can cause skin sensitivity. One of the most common and popular carrier oils is fractionated coconut oil. The term "fractionated" refers to a fraction of the coconut oil components being used in this application. This oil is a fraction of the whole, virgin coconut oil that is harvested.

Fractionation tends to prolong the oil's shelf life. Many vegetable oils can oxidize and spoil over time. Discard your oil if it smells rancid.

The dilution is typically a 1:3 ratio—one drop of essential oil to three drops of coconut oil. Dilution is very important when using essential oils. Don't worry—use of fractionated coconut oil or another carrier oil will not minimize the essential oil benefits. In fact, it makes the situation better by increasing the absorption and extending the benefits.

Although coconut oil is the most common carrier oil, it's not the only one. Any pure vegetable oil is a good carrier oil because these oils can easily dissolve an essential oil without disrupting the oil's effectiveness.

The following oils are also very commonly used as carrier oils because they are lightweight and non-greasy:

- Avocado oil
- Walnut oil
- Macadamia nut oil
- Sweet almond oil
- Linseed oil

- Sunflower oil
- Olive oil
- Apricot kernel oil
- Jojoba oil
- Grapeseed oil

Here are some examples of oils that always need to be diluted:

- Cassia
- Cinnamon
- Clove
- Cumin
- Geranium
- Lemongrass
- Oregano
- Thyme

You will typically find common carrier oils available for purchase in natural foods stores. It's preferable to buy carrier oils that are organic and cold-pressed. Most carrier oils do not have a strong smell, so they don't mask the scent of the essential oil you are using.

Ideally, keep your carrier oils refrigerated; they'll typically keep a year.

Topical use is a great essential oil application; since the VACs are so small, they easily pass through the skin into the bloodstream.

Skin

Many oils cleanse and purify and as such, have long been used to keep skin healthy. Oils are commonly used to soothe irritated skin and to help heal skin imperfections like acne.

Many modern skincare products contain chemicals, but essential oils are natural, free from fillers, chemicals and even toxins present in today's cleaners, toners and other skin products.

Oils can be used by people who have very sensitive skin who typically struggle to find a skincare product that won't cause a reaction. Instead, oils can simply be diluted to accommodate sensitive skin.

Lots of people make their own beauty and skin care remedies from essential oils. Here are a few ideas:

- Add geranium to your existing facial moisturizer. It will provide your skin with a healthy glow.
- Make your own body butter lotion with coconut oil, shea butter and essential oils.
- Use coconut oil, beeswax and lavender oil for a yummy and healing lip balm.
- Soothe your feet after a long day with a large basin of warm water and some lemon and eucalyptus oils.
- Some ladies swear by this cellulite remedy of coconut oil mixed with a few drops of grapefruit seed essential oil
- Create your own perfume with jasmine or ylang-ylang oil. Lavender and vanilla are great for women, and cypress and clove are great for men's natural chemistry.
- Make your own face wash with raw honey and tea tree oil. It's great for acne.
- Create a facial sugar scrub with sugar (or rock salt) and almond oil plus an essential oil of your choice.

- Make a natural skin toner with a cup of water, and two drops each of lavender, geranium and frankincense oils.
- To strengthen fingernails, use vitamin E and add lemon, frankincense and myrrh; rub on nails and cuticles
- Use sandalwood, geranium, lavender and frankincense essential oils with an unscented lotion as a great wrinkle reducer (avoid the eye area)
- Frankincense essential oil applied directly to sun spots and age spots can dramatically reduce their appearance
- Use coconut oil mixed with frankincense and myrrh and grapefruit seed essential oils to reduce stretch marks.
- Heal your dry, cracked feet by mixing coconut oil and lavender; apply to feet, wear socks overnight, and you'll wake up with soft and supple tootsies!

If you're going to have five oils on hand for skin and beauty, pick these:
- Calm irritated skin – lavender and Roman chamomile

- Reduce age spots – frankincense
- Thicken hair – rosemary and sage
- Natural SPF skin protection – helichrysum and myrrh
- Acne and blemishes - melaleuca (tea tree) and geranium

Body

Adding a few drops of oil to a warm bath can soak tired muscles and calm your senses. Lavender is a popular bath additive. Since oils are not water soluble, they'll float on top of the water, which is great for aromatherapy but not so great for skin absorption. Use a few tablespoons of whole milk or cream to act as a dispersant for the oil. This will ensure it is evenly spread throughout your bath water. Bath salts can also be used to disperse essential oils. Try this recipe: three parts sea salt, two parts Epsom salt and one part baking soda; add to that a few drops of your favorite oil.

Massage is one of the oldest topical uses of essential oil. You can massage body, feet, hands or any area that is sore and will benefit from massage. Therapists usually use about six drops of essential oil mixed with a carrier oil. Massaging the neck, forehead, temples, arms, legs, feet and hands with essential oils can be extremely relaxing.

If you sit for long hours at your desk, and you have tension in your neck and shoulders, consider an essential oils massage to unwind.

Some people apply oils topically to the chest to promote breathing and clear congestion.

Hot or cold compresses can be made by adding essential oils for their soothing properties.

If you've got sore muscles from a workout or joint pain from arthritis, you can use essential oils to soothe pain. Many oil manufacturers make oil pain blends. Many essential oils have cooling and warming properties, which help sore muscles.

You might have been instructed to apply oils on the bottoms of your feet. When first trying an oil, the bottom of the feet are a great starting point. The pores are larger, the skin is much thicker and less sensitive. Try it out! Lots of people place the oils on their feet prior to bedtime.

Have you ever had an upset stomach? Use a few drops of peppermint oil with coconut oil for a belly rub; it helps to calm your digestion and your upset stomach.

Hair

Adding essential oils to your hair products is a great way to provide extra moisture or deal with problems like an itchy, dry scalp. For example, rosemary can invigorate the scalp tissue. There are many hair care products on the market that already contain essential oils, such as argan oil for extra moisturizing.

Essential oils like lavender, sage and rosemary stimulate the scalp and hair follicles and can naturally thicken hair and help with hair loss. Hormone levels affect hair loss, and lavender and clary sage help to balance estrogen levels. Likewise, rosemary stops the hormone known as dihydroxy-testosteron or DHT, and therefore stops hair loss.

Here are some tried-and-true home remedies:
- A scalp massage oil made of 10 drops of rosemary oil and 5 drops of lavender oil
- A natural shampoo of coconut milk, aloe vera gel and lavender and rosemary oils

- Addition of lavender, cedarwood or basil essential oils to your shampoo to reduce itching
- A mix of unscented oil plus rosemary and lavender essential oils as a scalp massage for dandruff
- Rosemary oil added to shampoo to thicken hair and add volume
- Unscented oil mixed with sandalwood and lavender essential oils as a hair conditioner
- Ylang ylang, rosemary and lime oils mixed with unscented oil as a scalp massage for oily hair.

Gargle

Add essential oils to water to use as a gargle. Wintergreen and peppermint freshen breath and clove can help heal gums. In fact, when people develop a complication known as dry socket from wisdom tooth extraction surgery, a clove packet is put into the empty tooth socket. Patients feel immediate relief. Gargling with clove oil can have the same effect for inflamed gums. In fact, there are essential oil mouthwashes on the market; they contain a heavy amount of clove oil for gum healing. If you have a sore throat, gargle with tea tree oil. Whatever oil you use, it only takes a few drops in warm water. Do not swallow the gargle mixture.

Bug Spray

You can even make your own homemade, all natural bug spray and avoid chemicals like toxic DEET in commercial mosquito repellent products. All of the oils below repel insects. You can spray or rub them on to put insects at bay.

- Citronella
- Lemongrass
- Eucalyptus
- Peppermint
- Clove

Best Topical Oils

Here are just a few of the literally hundreds of topical uses for essential oils.

- Basil: Apply to the temples and neck to reduce tension
- Bergamot: Apply to the skin during your shower for skin-purifying benefits
- Black Pepper: Apply to your feet for a stimulating wake up
- Clary Sage: Apply to your abdomen during your menstrual cycle to help with cramps
- Roman Chamomile: Add to your favorite shampoo or conditioner
- Rose: Rub on face for even skin tone and healthy complexion
- Rosemary: Massage into the scalp
- Vetiver: Use for a foot massage after a long day of standing
- Mint oils (peppermint or wintergreen): place a few drops in hand, rub together, inhale for an energy boost

- Ylang Ylang: place on back of neck to calm and uplift

Topical Safety

For any topical product, you should always use safety precautions. Be sure to look for any irritation that occurs. Follow proper dosage, and use a carrier oil if recommended. Individuals react to essential oils differently, so it's wise to determine how your body will react to the new oil. Once you determine that, proceed with using these beneficial oils.

When essential oils are used topically, there is always the chance for sensitivity or skin irritation. Certain parts of your body, such as nasal tissues, mouth tissue, inner ears and eyes are very sensitive to oils. Be sure to wash your hands of excess oil, and avoid touching your face or rubbing your eyes if you have oil on your fingers.

Elderly people can have more skin sensitivity, particularly to high-menthol oils like eucalyptus and peppermint. The elderly may want to avoid certain oils or only use in a highly diluted form.

Here are oils known to cause skin irritation:

- Bay
- Cinnamon bark or leaf
- Clove bud
- Citronella
- Cumin
- Lemongrass
- Lemon verbena
- Oregano
- Thyme

The use of topical oils during pregnancy remains controversial. The main concern is for oils that can cross from the mother's body through the placenta to affect the baby. It's important to note that just because an oil crosses the placenta does not mean it will cause harm to either the mother or the fetus. Still, there are concerns, particularly about use of oils during the first trimester of pregnancy.

As an example, let's say a mother takes a nightly bath with a few drops of lavender for calming. While it is unlikely that this would cause any problems for the unborn child, use remains controversial.

It is an old wives' tale that use of oils like clary sage or rosemary in either an aromatherapy way or as a massage oil can cause a miscarriage. There are no recorded cases. Pregnant women have to take very large doses of essential oils like pennyroyal which then become a toxic dose.

Indeed, the occasional use of a few drops of safe oil as part of a bath or massage probably does more good than harm because it relaxes the mother and soothes the discomforts of pregnancy.

Still, there is lack of scientific information regarding oil use during pregnancy, so it is best to adhere to general safety guidelines regarding the oils and to check with your doctor prior to starting any use.

People with damaged, diseased, or inflamed skin are much more likely to be sensitive to oils and have skin reactions. Never use an undiluted oil on damaged or diseased skin because you may worsen the skin condition. Also, when skin is diseased, a larger than normal amount of oil might be absorbed.

Just remember that when it comes to topical use, it's better to use several small doses throughout the day rather than a single large dose. Small doses can be repeated every few hours.

Internal Ingestion

Certain essential oils can be ingested internally as dietary supplements. This is not a new concept; you essentially already do this—every time you have mint in your tea, cinnamon on your toast or basil on your pasta.

Because oils are in a concentrated form, they can be ingested to have targeted and potent effects on your health.

Internal use is safe and effective; once ingested, essential oils directly enter the blood stream through the gastrointestinal tract. Once there, they are transported throughout the rest of the body, and because they are soluble in lipids, all organs easily uptake and use them, including the brain.

Just like other nutrients we intake, oils are metabolized by the liver and then excreted as a waste product.

Proper dosing is particularly important when ingesting oils. Lots of oils users take essential oils internally in a veggie capsule or mix it with a bit of water or yogurt.

See the culinary uses of oil section for oils to use when cooking.

Ingestion Safety

The best rule of thumb is to never ingest an essential oil without professional advice from a practitioner or aromatherapist. A licensed individual will have certification from The Alliance of International Aromatherapists (AIA) or alternative agency. Just because someone sells essential oils does not mean they are a licensed professional, so beware.

The AIA does not endorse any internal use of oils unless recommended by a clinically trained health practitioner (doctor, nurse, etc.) for safety reasons.

Furthermore, there is not enough research on how essential oils interact with the gut's natural flora, meaning the roughly four pounds of healthy bacteria that lives in your digestive tract. It is unsure how each oil affects that bacteria and whether it contributes or detracts from the healthy flora balance.

There's no scientific support to say that essential oils only kill harmful bacteria; they may kill the beneficial gut bacteria too. Significantly more research is needed in this area.

Certainly, many oils have antibacterial qualities, but effects on gut bacteria are unknown at this time. There is some evidence to indicate that oils might be effective. Peppermint oil coated do help with inflammatory bowel disease; in one study, the oil did help the balance of beneficial gut bacteria.

Last but not least, for most oils, ingestion is not the most effective method. Ingestion is the right application only in very specific situations, so try to stick to aromatic and topical uses.

Oils have an effect on internal tissues and the delicate mucosal lining in the esophagus and other tissues, particularly in the digestive tract. Some studies show that certain oils, like citrus oils, contain limonene which might have a protective effect on mucosal tissues, but again, it is too early and there is not enough conclusive research, so erring on the side of caution is best.

Oils that should never be ingested internally are:

- Basil
- Birch
- Black pepper
- Cardamom
- Cedarwood
- Citronella
- Eucalyptus
- Melaleuca (Tea Tree)

How do I choose the best method to apply essential oils?

The application method chosen depends on the desired effect and the essential oil selected, but moreso, it depends on the labeled use of the oil, so follow those labels! For example, some essential oils are irritating to the skin because of their chemistry. These would need more dilution or might better be used by inhalation.

Here are some use tips:

- Topical applications are best for skin conditions and wound care.

- Use aromatherapy to lighten your mood.

- Taking a bath gives you a double dip, so to speak, since it involves topical absorption and aromatherapy.

If you're not sure how to use your new essential oils, consult a qualified aromatherapist.

What conditions can be treated with essential oils? Anxiety, depression, and stress

Aromatherapy is a real, effective therapy for mood disorders like depression and anxiety. Have you ever had chamomile tea at night to calm down? The essential oils of the plant are in the tea. They work, don't they? In a recent study conducted in China, scientists performed animal studies involving aromatherapy using Roman chamomile essential oil for two weeks. Amazingly, scientists used imaging to show the inhalation of the VACs "light up" in the hippocampus, the part of the animal's brain that regulates mood.

Certain essential oils like those in the mint family (spearmint, peppermint and others) contain the chemical compound carvone. Brazilian scientists published a recent study showing the significant calming effect of carvone on subjects with anxiety.

Anxiety is how your body prepares itself to deal with a threatening situation, and in today's stressful world, many experience some degree of anxiety, perhaps even on a daily basis. Over time, this form of stress takes its toll—emotionally and physically. Fear, nervousness and even palpitations are common symptoms. Heart rate and blood pressure both increase.

To soothe anxiety, here are the top essential oils to use:

- Lavender oil is considered a universal oil known for its relaxing effect. Mist your pillow before bedtime or add some to your bath.
- The fresh sharp scent of wild orange oil is very uplifting for both the body and the mind. It is also calming and has been shown to reducing heart palpitations brought on by anxiety.
- Lemon oil can lower blood pressure and calm nerves with its invigorating fragrance.
- Clary sage is actually part of the mint family, and mixed with bergamot oil, calms the nerves.
- Lemon balm helps people with the anxiety caused by an over-active thyroid.

Relaxation

Many of these same oils can be used for simple aromatherapy relaxation. Put a few drops of oil on your hands and rub them together to emit the wonderful smells. Or place oil on a cotton ball and breathe in the aroma. Massage therapists use essential oils during massage; not only are the oils absorbed through the skin, but their aroma is also released into the air for inhalation.

Insomnia

Who among us couldn't use a better night's sleep? Poor sleep has downstream repercussions on many other areas of health. For example, dementia patients are very prone to sleep disturbances. A Japanese study used aromatherapy for a 20-day period; oils were put onto a towel left near the patient's pillow. Subjects slept longer and got better quality of sleep.

Single oils like lavender and chamomile are very effective for sleep, and there are also blended oils designed for sleep that contain lavender, chamomile, and other oils such as cedarwood or vetiver. Here are the best sleep-inducing oils:

- Lavender is most known for being related to sleep. It can be used in a diffuser or as a mist on your pillow. It is so effective that hospital ICUs are starting to use it to help patients sleep.

- Vetiver essential oil is distilled from the roots of the plant, so it has a rich, earthy smell. If you want your brain to shut off for a good night's sleep, this is your oil.

- Roman chamomile is best known for its tea possessing calming, soothing, and relaxing properties. Chamomile oil's light, floral scent will get you at peace in no time.

- Ylang Ylang has a fruity and floral scent that can help the quality of your sleep.

- Bergamot is a citrus fruit often added to teas. Bergamot is described as emotional balancing and will definitely help you sleep.

Allergy

Essential oils might be useful in seasonal allergy symptoms. Oils used for respiratory support contain the chemical compound eucalyptol, shown to be very effective in combating the immune system changes that occur with seasonal allergies. Oregano has long been used for respiratory problems, and other oils like cardamom and rosemary are very effective. In a recent study in mice, essential oil compound mixtures showed a great reduction in airway inflammation.

An allergy is an abnormal response by your immune system when it comes into contact with a specific substance known as an allergen. Your body releases histamine for allergens like food, grasses and pollens, mold and pet hair. Essential oils are a great all-natural alternative to medications. Here are the top five:

- Melaleuca (Tea Tree) – to treat mold and fungi allergies.

- Roman Chamomile – great for respiratory problems stemming from allergies.
- Melissa (Lemon Balm) – Melissa is from the mint family and this oil can be inhaled to easy any allergic reaction
- Peppermint – this oil can be applied directly to the skin or diluted to help with pollen and other seasonal allergies. The L-menthol in the oil stops inflammation.
- Lavender – lavender can halt immediate allergic reactions that result in swelling or itching.

Immune System

Our immune systems suffer a daily onslaught of bacteria, viruses and environmental threats. Add in lifestyle factors of stress and poor sleep, and our immune systems usually do not fare well. Immunity has two parts. The first line of defense protects the body from invader entry; the skin and gastrointestinal tract are good examples. If an invader does happen to get past the first line of defense, we have mobilized immunity that comes to the rescue. White blood cells rush to the infection. Boosting both aspects of the immune system is important in order to stay healthy.

Oregano is powerful for respiratory issues. Clove oil has both anti-bacterial and anti-parasite qualities. A protein called chitin is produced by insects as a waste product. People inhale it from the circulating air. Chitin is an example of one of the intruders we are exposed to on a daily basis. Scientists studied the effects of peppermint and thyme essential oils on chitin. Amazingly, these oils reversed the negative respiratory effects of chitin. The chitin is still present in the air—nothing can be done about that—but the oils made the cells not have an adverse reaction to it.

You're probably tempted to run and get antibiotics every time you get a cold, but that won't work because viruses—not bacteria—cause colds. There's no cure for a cold—you just have to tough it out. Rest and stay hydrated. But there are some oils you can add to diffuse through the air, and that might help:

- Eucalyptus has both antibacterial and antiviral properties and is part of many over-the-counter products because of it. It helps to dilate the bronchioles for easy breathing and it can break up the mucus of congestion. Use it if you have congestion or a stuffy nose or cough.

- Cardamom helps ease any stomach upset you might have with the cold.

- Geranium flowers may smell great but the oil also has tremendous antiseptic and antibacterial properties. It's great for disinfecting the air and surfaces in your home, which is very helpful when you have a sick household.

- Lemon is great to have around the house for so many reasons, but it can be particularly effective during illness. Your lymphatic system becomes sluggish when you're ill and this oil can mildly stimulate the lymphatics.

- Peppermint, like cardamom, can soothe stomachs and reduce nausea. It is also great for coughs. It's a real immune-booster.

- Rosemary is mostly known for cooking but it is very helpful for a cough and joint pains that often happen when you have a cold. It also zaps headaches.

Arthritis and Joint Pain

Essential oils can be topically applied right to the muscle or joint to relieve pain. Some of these oils require a carrier oil to help the oil go deep into the tissue. The oils are rapidly absorbed through the skin, so they're a very effective method and natural, anti-inflammatory agent at site of the inflammation that is caused by arthritis.

Several research studies have shown that topical essential oils can be effective against arthritis. Here are the most effective oils.

- Ginger has amazing healing agents that are both analgesic and anti-inflammatory. It decreases pain associated with arthritis by acting on the vanilloid receptors of the sensory nerves. When applied, the ginger oil can have a slight burning sensation, so a carrier oil is recommended. The Arthritis Foundation reported on a study that showed ginger can even substitute for nonsteroidal anti-inflammatory drugs (NSAIDs) like Tylenol. Research has shown that ginger affects inflammation at the cellular level, making it a great option for arthritis sufferers.

- Turmeric, also called curcumin, is known as a great anti-inflammatory agent and has been shown to be highly effective, particularly for people managing rheumatoid arthritis (RA). Turmeric acts on a chemical called interleukin (IL)-6, which causes the inflammation specific to RA. Patients take turmeric veggie caps and drink turmeric tea and smoothies.

- Frankincense is a very old oil. It's so old that it is mentioned in the Old Testament. Researchers know that it inhibits the body's production of key inflammatory molecules specific to conditions like arthritis. Frankincense can also help prevent the breakdown of cartilage tissue in the joints, the main cause of arthritis pain. It's truly a natural treatment option for pain-related conditions of the muscles, joints and tendons.

- Myrrh oil is another ancient oil like frankincense. It also has anti-inflammatory properties, and is often used together with frankincense to treat arthritis. Together, the oils suppress the intensity of inflammation in the joints.

- Orange oil also has strong anti-inflammatory properties. Orange oil had the highest level of antioxidants, which makes it a great essential oil for arthritis treatment. Use avocado or almond oil as a carrier oil, then rub into joints wherever you have pain.

Inflammation

More people than ever are suffering from rampant inflammation, which wreaks havoc on so many body systems. Over time, chronic inflammation has drastic effects. The human body is supposed to naturally regulate inflammation, but immune systems are so under fire from stress, pollutants and other factors that many people have inflammation that is out of control. Certain oils like thyme and oregano have a compound called carvacrol that supports the immune system. A group of scientists in 2015 found that carvacrol kept the body from overproducing the inflammatory molecules that lead to negative effects.

Visible inflammation causes pain, redness, immobility, swelling and heat. Yet there are many types of chronic inflammation inside the body which we cannot see. Here are the best oils to help you fight inflammation.

- Peppermint is great for reducing the acute inflammation caused by injury, and can be even more effective when used with lavender and German chamomile in an anti-inflammatory blend.

- Eucalyptus works well on respiratory inflammation--bronchitis, laryngitis, pneumonia. It packs a punch as an anti-inflammatory, antibacterial, decongestant and mucolytic (breaks up mucus). It works well with spruce and spike lavender in a respiratory essential oil blend.

- And speaking of lavender, it also is effective on respiratory inflammation, but also works well in infections and acute inflammation due to injury.

- German chamomile is particularly effective for inflammatory skin conditions

- Spruce oil eases the pain in arthritis or swollen joints. It has analgesic and anti-inflammatory properties.

Healing

Several oils fit the bill to promote general healing:

- Arnica Oil: arnica has long been added to natural pain reliever products. It has natural anti-inflammatory properties and has been shown in research studies to be useful in treating osteoarthritis as well as carpal tunnel syndrome. It's great for acute sports-related injuries.

- Basil oil can really help if you are fighting a cold or allergies. The oil is high in antioxidants and has both antibacterial and antifungal properties. People use it to treat everything from ear infections to urinary tract infections.

- Tea tree oil does so many things. It is extremely versatile and a must-have for any medicine cabinet. It is useful for bacterial infections, insect bites, cold sores, earaches, and even psoriasis. It has tremendous antimicrobial.

- Lavender can induce sleep, which is very important for healing. It is easily the most popular essential oil for its many uses. Lavender can be helpful in diabetes management because it balances blood sugar.
- Peppermint oil is really effective against several types of digestive disorders, like indigestion or irritable bowel syndrome.
-

Energy Boost

Who doesn't need an energy boost, practically daily? Here are a few oils you may not realize can give you that much-needed energy boost.

- Basil: There are two types of basil essential oil, exotic basil and French (sweet) basil. French basil is the only one safe to use in aromatherapy; besides, it smells better. Basil oil is known to stimulate the adrenal glands, releasing hormones that help fight mental fatigue. Basil is often blended with lime, spearmint and rosemary.

- Ginger essential oil has an invigorating effect on nerves, and can pep you up even if you got no sleep. It is often blended with lime essential oil.

- Speaking of lime, this essential oil is a great restorative. Use it if you've had trouble concentrating. It blends well with basil, ginger, and rosemary.

- Mint oils like peppermint and spearmint do act similarly. Spearmint is the milder of the two. It can have a tremendous calming effect on the nervous system.

- Rosemary essential oil is a stimulant, and can give you that boost you sorely need. People use it when mental fatigue or low energy set in.

Digestion

More and more, we're learning that a healthy digestive system is foundational to good health. Many Americans have gut issues and are looking for a natural way to restore their gastrointestinal comfort and normal digestion. Look no further than essential oils:

Peppermint has long been associated with soothing stomach aches and providing gastrointestinal comfort. It supports healthy gut bacteria and makes digestion more efficient.

Pregnancy and childbirth

For thousands of years, midwives have used essential oils to ease the pain of pregnancy and delivery. Modern midwives still use these oils for massage, and patients report less anxiety and pain.

Always check with your midwife or doctor before you use oils during pregnancy. Many oils affect hormone levels and alter your body's functions. For example, peppermint oil is known to decrease milk supply in nursing mothers. Clary sage should only be used by a midwife during labor.

Here are some other oils to avoid while pregnant and nursing: *aniseed, angelica, basil, birch, black pepper, camphor, cinnamon, chamomile, clary sage, clove, cypress, fennel, fir, ginger, hyssop, jasmine, juniper, marjoram, myrrh, nutmeg, oak moss, oregano, parsley seed, pennyroyal, peppermint, rose, rosemary, rue, sage, tarragon, thyme, wintergreen and wormwood.*

The following oils are generally safe during pregnancy, used according to proper dilution methods: *benzoin, bergamot, black pepper, chamomile (German & Roman), clary sage, cypress, eucalyptus, frankincense, geranium, ginger, grapefruit, juniper, lavender, lemon, mandarin, majoram (sweet), neroli, petitgrain, rose, sandalwood, orange (sweet), tea tree, ylang ylang.*

Buying Guide

It is really important to have proper knowledge about buying essential oils. They typically come in 5ml, 10ml and 15ml bottles. Some of the rarer and more expensive oils might be sold in 1ml and 2ml sizes.

The U.S. FDA does not regulate essential oils, so finding a quality distributor is imperative.

Not all essential oils are created equal. There are many worthless products on the market. You'll find many synthetic products, too.

There are four things you want to look for:

- USDA organic certification
- 100 percent pure labeling
- Therapeutic grade oils
- Indigenously sourced oils
- Labeling regarding whether the oil has been diluted

For starters, comparison shop for several brands of the same oil. Most likely the really inexpensive ones are probably diluted, synthetic or made with cheaper ingredients, and not worth your money. Low prices are red flags, unless the company is offering a promotional discount.

Legitimate sellers are transparent about describing their products. Their websites should have quality control documents you can download about the contents of their oils and how they make their product.

Look at the ingredients. Legitimate sellers should list all the ingredients.

Therapeutic grade oils are the highest grade. Wellness grade oils are the next grade and indicate a steam-distilled product; the source plants may have been sprayed with pesticides. Just because an oil says "pure", doesn't mean it is quality. This is the most common form of labeling and the most commonly sold essential oil; normally the oils are over-processed. The lowest grade consists of synthetic and altered oils that have been created in a lab.

Always buy therapeutic grade oils. They're made of the highest quality plants and grown in organic soil. They've been made by steam distillation or cold-pressing without the use of chemicals.

The cost of an essential oil is determined by several factors, including the plant used, the method of production, and the quantity of oil to be produced.

Citrus oils are reasonably affordable whereas rose, jasmine and sandalwood are very costly.

There are subtypes of essential oil, all referred to under the blanket term "essential oil" because they're all natural, concentrated, liquid aromatics, just obtained by different methods.

- Absolutes: made from rare botanicals like jasmine and rose, solvent extraction is used to obtain the precious oil.

- CO_2 Extracts: CO_2-extracted oils use carbon dioxide as a solvent. The CO_2 is converted to liquid under low temperature, high pressure conditions. The active components and oils of the plant are then collected in the cool liquid. When extraction is complete, the carbon dioxide is reverted to its gaseous form. Left behind are the essential oils.

It is important to remember that essential oils and fragrance oils are definitely not the same things. Essential oils are the true aromatic essence of the plant and are highly concentrated. Furthermore, essential oils are usually not referred to as fragrances.

Fragrance oils are usually listed as just "fragrance" in an ingredient list. These oils are generally synthetic and therefore much less expensive than essential oils.

Typically available in hundreds of scents, many products can be created with fragrance oils that mimic natural essential oils scents.

Because they're synthetic, fragrance oils are much more likely to cause allergies or skin irritation in individuals who use them. This is the very reason why many people opt for perfume-free products like laundry detergent and lotions. Essential oils are considered much less gentle.

Just because a product contains a fragrance oil doesn't mean it is of inferior quality. Its use is often a trade-off in cost. When manufacturers make candles or soaps, it takes a lot more essential oil to create the fragrance. That is why many products are all natural, such as beeswax candles or soap, except for the fragrance.

To tell the difference, just know that products with fragrance oils are not allowed to be listed as being 100% natural, because they're not. The fragrances are synthetic. A fragrance oil may be listed as "lavender fragrance" while an essential oil containing product will be listed as *Lavandula officinalis* (lavender oil).

How to store essential oils

Most essential oils come in dark glass containers to keep light out since light and UV rays can change the oils by creating oxidation. Store oils in a cool place. Once opened, most oils can be safely used for one to two years.

Essential oils typically do not become rancid, but they do oxidize and therefore lose their beneficial properties. Citrus oils are particularly susceptible to oxidation, sometimes losing their effectiveness in as little as six months.

Other oils mature with age, like patchouli and sandalwood.

Properly store oils in dark brown or blue bottles; these dark glasses shield the oils from sunlight, which can deteriorate the oils. It's the same reason why most bottled beers are stored in brown bottles. It is unwise to store your oils in clear bottles or plastic bottles. Some oils will degrade the plastic and ruin the oil in a short amount of time.

Some vendors sell oils in aluminum bottles, which is fine as long as the bottles are lined so the oil does not interact with the metal.

Also try not to purchase essential oils with a rubber dropper as a cap. Always buy oils with a screw top cap. The dropper should be separate as the oil will degrade the rubber. Rather than a dropper bottle, it is acceptable to purchase small bottles with a top called an orifice reducer, which is a small, clear insert that fits inside the bottle to serve as a built-in dropper. To use it, tip the bottle to dispense the oil drops. The reducers are made of materials that stand up to any oil. If your oils come with the orifice reducers, it is one indication that you are purchasing a high-quality oil.

Always store oils in a cool, dark place, such as a wooden box with a lid. Better yet, refrigerate your oils if possible.

Essential Oil Starter Kit

If you could purchase just 10 well-rounded oils, what would they be? Here is a suggestion of a top 10 list.

- Bergamot's citrusy aroma is great for healing skin and lifting moods

- Clove oil is perfect for pain relief and inflammation and great for inflamed gum tissues

- Eucalyptus oil is a great decongestant and topical pain reliever

- Frankincense has anti-microbial and anti-inflammatory properties and is one of the oldest oils in the world

- Lavender is calming and sleep-inducing

- Lemon oil is anti-fungal and an all-around household cleaner and air freshener

- Oregano helps skin conditions like eczema and psoriasis

- Peppermint aids digestion and eases headaches

- Rosemary detoxifies and helps skin and hair, and you can cook with it!

- Tea tree (melaleuca) helps skin and scalp

The Best Oils To Have In Your Medicine Cabinet

What if you could build a medicine cabinet just out of essential oils? What would you choose? You'd need headache relief, insect sting remedies and sunburn relief. Here is a recommendation for a natural essential oil medicine cabinet without the side effects of conventional drugs like aspirin and antibiotics.

- Lavender for cuts, stings, burns, and rashes. It also reduces anxiety and helps you fall asleep.
- Peppermint helps headaches and muscle and joint pain. It also helps with digestive issues

and asthma and bronchitis. This wonder oil can also reduce fever and clear sinuses.

- Frankincense is a powerful anti-inflammatory agent with all sorts of uses.
- Melaleuca (tea tree) is both an antibacterial and antifungal. It can reduce or even prevent infection and can clean the air of allergens.

- You may want to also have some eucalyptus, oregano and clove on hand. Oregano acts like an antibiotic, and the others have multiple remedies.

Essential Oils for Weight Loss

You may have heard about people using essential oils for weight loss, and there are some oils that can help. Keep in mind that the oils just help with weight loss. They are not a cure all. Dietary changes and exercise are the mainstays, but oils can provide an extra boost to help you reach a weight loss goal. The oils are much more natural than caffeine and other stimulants. These four oils help support fat loss:

- Peppermint oil suppresses cravings and improves digestion

- Grapefruit oil contains the compound d-limonene found in citrus peels. D-limonene improves metabolic enzyme levels which speeds up your metabolism.
- Cinnamon bark oil helps to balance blood sugar levels. When those levels are balanced, weight loss is easier.
- Ginger oil contains gingerol, which decreases inflammation and increases thermogenesis, turning each cell into a fat burning factory that boosts metabolism.

Best Essential Oil Remedies

When you look at this long list of remedies, it is clear to see that essential oils have some incredible properties.

- Migraine headache relief
- Reduce cough or sinus pressure
- Heal burns
- Soothe bug bites
- Improve digestion
- Bronchitis and asthma remedy
- Treat bruises
- Improve concentration
- Sore feet soak
- Reduce teeth grinding
- Relieve PMS
- Eczema and psoriasis cream
- Improve circulation
- Relieve hangover symptoms
- Curb food cravings
- Energize your workout
- Reduce fever
- Relieve motion sickness

- Arthritis relief
- Treat ringworm
- Head lice treatment
- Heal blistered skin
- Soothe a sunburn
- Treat poison oak
- Lose weight
- Boost immune system
- Sore muscles
- Reduce morning sickness
- Improve allergies
- Kick a cold
- Reduce back and neck pain

Home Uses

Essential oils can be used throughout the home to support wellness through a clean environment.

- First, lemon is a powerful all-purpose cleaner that leaves a fresh, clean scent. It is a natural disinfectant. Add a few drops of tea tree for an added boost.

- Spray your kids sports gear with a mixture of the lemon/tea tree with four tablespoons of baking soda added to warm water. It will definitely disinfect and de-funkify those ripe-smelling uniforms and shoes.

- Cinnamon is a natural anti-microbial that is great sprayed in the air.

- Add 20 drops of your favorite oil to every laundry load, and it will not only make those clothes and sheets smell great, it will keep your washing machine smelling great too.

- Add some drops of any oil to your vacuum cleaner and it won't smell dusty any more.

- You can make your own sunscreen from essential oils. Just mix coconut oil with some zinc oxide and shea butter, then add lavender and helichrysum oils. Mix together and store in a squeeze bottle. You'll be sun free and toxin free too.

- Every home has had yucky shower curtain scum from time to time. Fill a spray bottle with warm water and add four drops each of eucalyptus and tea tree essential oils and you'll have a natural mold-killer that will get rid of the scum. Add tea tree oil to your diffuser to kill mold and other pathogens in the air.

- Who hasn't experienced a burnt-bottom kitchen pan at one time or another? Never fear. Just add some water and lemon oil and boil.

- Have a great smelling home by diffusing a blend of orange, clove and rosemary. Your house will smell amazing. Guests will comment.

- You can make your own homemade carpet freshening powder out of borax and 20 drops of tea tree oil.

- Don't use harsh pesticides. Make a mixture of orange and clove oils and spray your pest. It will be killed on contact.

- Add a couple of drops of lemon oil to a bowl of water and wash all your fruit and vegetables

- A clove, cinnamon and citrus essential oil mixture in a simmering pan of water will get rid of cooking odors

- Combine a half cup each of vinegar and baking soda with bergamot or lime oil and use it to scrub your sink or tub.

- To freshen your trash can place a cotton ball soaked in lemon oil to cut down of trash odor. You can do the same and place a cotton ball behind your toilet.

- Rinse your refrigerator with a water mixture containing lime, grapefruit or bergamot oil

- Make a blend of eucalyptus, tea tree and rosemary oils to eliminate cigar or cigarette smoke from your home.

- Add lemon oil to your dishwasher. You'll have cleaner spot-free dishes and a great smelling dishwasher

Industrial Uses

Essential oils have long been used in industrial cleaning products. If you smell that lemon furniture polish or that almond-scented floor cleaner, chances are it contains an essential oil. Many pest control products contain oils like citronella. Vicks Vaporub has eucalyptus oil.

Hospital Use

Hospitals are using oils for aromatherapy and to reduce infections. Vanderbilt University Hospital, for example, regularly uses the oils to treat depression and anxiety, but also to reduce infections.

Research studies show that patients who did lavender aromatherapy prior to surgery were less anxious about it.

Midwives also use specific essential oils to reduce fear and anxiety during labor. Essential oils can also have antibacterial or antifungal benefits and can be used to keep equipment clean.

Hospitals are definitely catching on to essential oils, using them to treat burns, as a sleep aid, for massage and to boost the immune system.

There are even studies underway to determine whether certain essential oils like frankincense can help fight cancer.

Veterinary Uses

Essential oils can absolutely be used in veterinary applications on animals. In fact, the use of synthetic repellents for fleas and other pests is becoming very problematic. Animals, like humans, develop sensitivities or allergic reactions. A blend of citronella, lemon and eucalyptus essential oils has been used with success, and citronella, clove and lily of the valley oils have been effective against ticks—just as effective in fact as the chemical DEET, but without all the toxic side effects.

Dogs and cats suffer from several fungal skin conditions that cause excessive itching. A blend of essential oils (lavender, bitter orange, oregano, marjoram, peppermint and helichrysum) with carriers, coconut oil and sweet almond oil, proved effective. In the study, animals treated for one month with the oil blend fared the same as the medicated control group.

Tea tree oil has been used effectively to fight mites. Tea tree oil is very toxic to pets unless used in the right concentrations by a trained veterinarian. The Journal of the American Veterinary Association reported hundreds of incidents of tea tree oil toxicity in pets in a 10 year period. Dogs and cats cannot tolerate pure tea tree oil in the same concentration that a human can.

In the same way, aromatherapy may have adverse effects on your pets for the same reasons. Larger animals tolerate it well. In fact, there have even been research studies showing lavender's effectiveness on horses by keeping them calm.

Veterinarians on commercial farms are also putting essential oils into practice. Many farmers are adding the oils to food to keep their intestinal health strong and to fight infections. Farmers who are raising antibiotic-free poultry say that they regularly use oregano oil and cinnamon oil to fight infection on farms. It has an amazing effect on gut bacteria in the animals. The oregano oil kills the bad bacteria and cinnamon oil supports the good bacteria.

Culinary Uses

Food is central to all world cultures. It's always present in times of celebration. So many people around the world love to cook; great cooks are always looking for new herbs, spices and flavor combinations.

Have you ever thought about cooking with essential oils? Lots of great cooks do. In fact, you likely already do, too, without realizing it. Every time you add olive oil or avocado oil to a dish, you're cooking with essential oils.

However, you may not have tried oils as flavoring agents, but you should. You'll be surprised at how the addition of one or two drops of oil adds flare to a recipe. Just remember that there is a significant

So, the idea that cooking with essential oils or incorporating them into our kitchen process is nothing new. The important thing is to do it safely, appreciating the differences between a whole herb or spice and its essential oil.

You'll also want to note that not every essential oil is a good choice for cooking. Sometimes cooking with essential oils doesn't taste quite as yummy as the whole herb.

Cooking with essential oils is pretty easy and it adds so much flavor to food. How great would it be to just add two drops of oil instead of all that chopping?

Because essential oil is so concentrated, you're using a much smaller portion when you cook. There's not a one-size-fits-all rule for how to convert whole herbs to oil, but in general, one drop of oil is equal to one teaspoon of chopped fresh or dried herbs or spices.

When you cook with an oil, you're going to use a similar carrier oil concept. Always dilute your drops of essential oil into a fat—olive oil, coconut oil, chicken fat, butter—whatever your recipe calls for. The fat helps disperse the oil into the entire dish so it's not just concentrated in one area.

If you're making a dessert, you can disperse the oil into syrup or honey. If you're creating a hot dish, add the essential oil at the very end of the cooking process. Remember they're volatile and they'll burn off easily, especially under high heat. Most cooks remove the dish from the heat, then stir in the diluted oil.

Cooks are sometimes hesitant to use essential oils because they feel that the heat damages the oil's properties, in particular by evaporation or alteration of the oil's chemical structures. It can happen, but the best way to prevent it is to minimize heat exposure.

Just remember that when you cook with essential oils, it's not so much that you're using the oil for health benefits. Rather, you're adding the oil for flavor and aroma of the dish.

Here are 10 staple oils you should have in your kitchen:

- Lavender is a very gentle oil with a delicate flavor for desserts and fish. You can even flavor lemonade with it.
- Peppermint is cool and refreshing in tea, lemonade and lots of desserts, especially chocolate ones.

- Citrus oils are great for cooking and you can use them in almost anything from smoothies to stir-fry.

- Bergamot is a citrus, but it is different. It's not a fruit that is normally eaten so its oil essence is a special treat in tea and scones.

- Cinnamon is most known for cookie flavoring, but it excellent in any sweet dish.

- Cardamom pairs well with cinnamon and is the flavor you taste when you drink chai. Cardamom can be used in any dessert that calls for spices and is also good on meat.

- Ginger root is used in gingerbread, stir fry and lots of marinades.

- Thyme is a favorite culinary herb that is good in meat dishes, soups and stews. It's excellent on poultry.

- Anise is famous for its licorice flavor, and can be added to any kind of cookie, but is great in marinades and soups too. Anise has a similar flavor to fennel and is good on meat, chicken or fish.

- Coriander/cilantro are from the same plant. Coriander is the seed and cilantro is the leaf.

Their flavors are drastically different. Cilantro oil can be added to salsas, while coriander oil goes great in savory dishes, sauces and vegetable dishes.

What Does Research Say?

Even though essential oils have been used for medical remedies for thousands of years, there is still very little published research on the topic. But that is beginning to change, as the potential power of essential oils is becoming more evident. Studies are going on around the world, in countries like Europe, Australia, Japan, India, the United States, and Canada.

The research is certainly being done by industries, like the food and cosmetics industries, but also by agricultural outlets looking for a non-antibiotic way to raise livestock. They're looking at flavoring that can be provided by essential oils, but also looking at its food preservative qualities as well as adding it to livestock food. Some companies are conducting extensive research on toxicity and safety.

Since it is corporate research, much of it is under wraps, but it is starting to make its way into scientific journals. Results are promising. It is important for scientists to keep adding to journals to grow our body of knowledge on essential oils. It's important to say that many studies to date have been animal studies and have not been conducted on humans, but that is taking shape as the research progresses.

Here are some of the issues that researchers have pointed out.

- Essential oils are not standardized. Plant chemistry is affected by local growing conditions and weather, as well as harvest time and season. As such, no two oils are exactly the same, unlike pharmaceutical drugs that are reproduced to be identical. If you alter an essential oil to make it standard, then it is no longer natural.

- There are not enough blind studies. The oils are so fragrant, you can't hide what you're studying. People associate smells with past experiences, so these studies are difficult to execute.

- There is not much funding of essential oil research. There are not many who want to sponsor research that doesn't follow a conventional clinical research approach of testing in the lab, then animals then humans. Most researchers want to jump straight to testing on humans because of oils' long history and known safety. The pharmaceutical industry funds most of these studies; they're not motivated to fund research that will directly compete with their conventional products.

- It is difficult to determine the study outcome. For example, oils are used in massage. Was the outcome due solely to the oil, to the massage or to both? Furthermore, essential oils are composed of hundreds of chemicals and it is hard to determine the active one or ones.

Despite these concerns, research does appear promising, and shows positive effects in a whole host of areas, including infections, pain, anxiety, depression, tumors, premenstrual syndrome and nausea.

Common Misconceptions About Essential Oils

In closing, let's dispel the most common myths about essential oils. It's important to separate fact from fiction for a clear picture of the benefits of these oils going forward.

Myth: Specific oils are the only ways to treat certain conditions.

There is no "one oil, one ailment" mantra. Certainly you must keep the ailment or condition in mind, but there are multiple oil solutions to a particular issue. Always remember--there are many paths to wellness.

Myth: You should take essential oils every day for disease prevention.

You don't take something every day in case you get a toothache, so you likely don't need to take essential oils every day unless you need something. Good holistic practices will get you pretty far in life. Taking or inhaling a certain oil every day won't guarantee you won't get sick, but they will certainly help.

Myth: Essential oils can't be used on pets.

Many vets are treating pets with essential oils. Just know that certain oils might be toxic because pets will not tolerate the oils as humans do. Talk to your vet about using aromatherapy around pets to determine its safety. In particular, cats might be susceptible to essential oils because they lack a liver enzyme that other animals have, therefore substances might be more toxic to cats because they can't process it.

Myth: Essential oils must always be blended and can only be used topically.

Both of these are false. Oils can be used topically, in aromatherapy and even ingested. They do not always have to be diluted for use either. Some can be used full strength.

Myth: Essential oils expire

Essential oils don't expire. If not stored in brown bottles, they can be affected by light exposure which can limit their shelf life. Some age well over time. Many people use expired therapeutic oils for cleaning applications.

Myth: Essential oils are only useful for therapeutic reasons.

Absolutely false. As you've read in this book, oils are used for a variety of important functions on our planet. Aromatherapy is definitely in the mainstream as a healing art, and it's good to be recognized in that way, but essential oils have many applications, including culinary, agricultural and industrial. The sky is the limit as researchers and companies unlock the great potential of essential oils.

Summary

Although oils like frankincense have been used for thousands of years, we are on the cusp of the next great research revelation in finding out about more essential oils and the positive effects they have on the human body. The near future will be an exciting new era as researchers embark upon this journey to determine what essential oils truly are, and more importantly, what they're not.

If you enjoyed learning about essential oils from this bundle, I would be forever grateful if you could leave a review on Amazon. Reviews are by far the best way to help newer authors, like myself, out. It also helps your fellow readers sort through and find the good books so make sure to help them out. Thanks so much in advance for your review!

www.ingramcontent.com/pod-product-compliance
Lightning Source LLC
Chambersburg PA
CBHW031120020426
42333CB00012B/155